The Wisdom of Fairy Tales

Born in 1896 in Hanover, Germany, Rudolf
Meyer studied theology, philosophy and Germanic languages before becoming a priest in
the newly-founded Christian Community. He
worked in Breslau and Prague, the Ruhr dis-
trict, during the war in Zurich, and later in
Karlsruhe. A prolific writer he has covered such
diverse subjects as education, the Grail, the
Gospels, and mythology, in over thirty books.
He died in 1986.

Rudolf Meyer

The Wisdom of Fairy Tales

Floris Books
Anthroposophic Press

Translated by Polly Lawson

Originally published in German under the title
Die Weisheit der deutschen Volksmärchen
by Verlag Urachhaus, Stuttgart.
Translated from the eighth German edition (1981).
This translation first published by Floris Books in 1988.
This paperback edition published in 1995.

British Library CIP Data available

ISBN 0-86315-208-2

Printed in Great Britain
by Cromwell Press, Wilts

Contents

Grimms' fairy tales

This book refers extensively to Grimm's fairy tales. In English there are two translations available. The older, *The Complete Grimm's Fairy Tales,* was published in 1944 by Pantheon Books (republished in the United States by Random Books, in Britain by Routledge & Kegan Paul). The newer, *The Complete Grimm's Tales for Young and Old,* was translated by Ralph Mannheim and published in America by Doubleday in 1977, and in Britain by Victor Gollancz in 1978 (republished by Penguin). The latter appears to be accurate and in more current English. The few quotations in this volume are taken from this translation.

1

The inner meaning
of fairy-tales

We cannot imagine a springtime without snowdrops, violets or primroses. We love them as the very idea of spring. If we were ever to become indifferent to their flowering, it would be a sure sign that in our hearts we had broken faith with the earth. It is equally impossible to imagine a childhood without Snow White, Little Red Riding Hood or the Frog King. Our unfolding sensibilities were nourished by them, and the fairy-tale princes seemed more real than the strange adults about us. What these colourful characters suffered, desired and achieved meant more to us than the assumed gravity which adults seemed to attach to everyday things.

The characters in the fairy-tales led us to discover the treasures in our own souls. We became instinctively aware of the sorrows of life and the guidance of destiny. Through them we learned that faithfulness makes the soul beautiful, that purity is the soul's highest joy and that only in poverty does its inmost radiance begin to shine. Through these characters we understood and accepted much against which our minds, blunted and mulish in later years, began to rebel.

We were able to appreciate that Thousandfurs had to undergo the deepest humiliation before she could break open the nutshells to reveal the shining dresses, and that we must at some time risk our life to win a princess. It became clear that we were born on earth just because there were so many wonderful adventures waiting for us.

Fairy-stories told and retold by mother to child enrich those depths of soul from which our later hopes and ideals are born. Millions of human souls absorb the fairy-tale motifs during their formative years, and their feelings are given a direction which influences the whole character of a people. No other literary creation, not even the most lofty classical work, has such a fundamental effect on generations of people.

While philosophies, artistic styles and religious conventions have changed over the centuries, the fairy-tales and their basic motifs have endured through the rise and fall of nations. However, during the eighteenth century, when reason entered upon her sovereign rule in questions of taste and belief, the folk-tale was scorned and left with simple people in spinning-rooms and quiet corners of the village. How proud were the "enlightened" as they gazed down from the heights into the depths of superstition. Of course animals could not speak or princes become bears or lions, and there were no dragons laying the country to waste and devouring maidens. Life had been placed on a reliable bourgeois footing where the world moved strictly in accordance with the laws of nature; this was the victory of modernity over the "Dark Ages".

Goethe and the younger generation of Romantics are to be thanked for breaking the tyranny of this "enlightened" bourgeois arrogance. Goethe gave expression in new fairy-tales to his soul's deepest experience. Novalis, Brentano, Mörike and others followed him; for them the fairy-tale is not an arbitrary play of fantasy or the fortuitous result of folk imagination, but as Novalis said, "the genuine fairy-tale must appear prophetic, idealistic and inevitable, all in one."

Is it not possible for us to discover this inner kingdom of the soul where in a new order of things we are all kings and will, one day, inherit kingdoms? For it is in this inner soul realm that the fairy-tale characters lead their lives in eternal youth and, heedless of the rigid laws of nature, pass through their transformations.

What took place in the course of evolution is repeated in some form as a stage in the life of each individual. Western man reached his "earth maturity" only with the coming of the age of discovery, of scientific investigation and the liberation of his personal and private life from the dictates of the Church. The spiritual struggles of the sixteenth to nineteenth centuries are reflected in the experience of adolescence. As the intellect awakes the young person begins to question tradition and authority. He experiences this new-found freedom by "protesting" and tests his own strength by rejecting all working of grace. He is now "enlightened". Before the eye of his soul the land of fairy and all its inhabitants grow pale.

While she is still in the cradle, the fate of the king's daughter is foretold: when she is fifteen, the princess will prick her finger on a spindle and fall down dead. However hard we may try to destroy all the spindles in the kingdom, Brier Rose, when her day comes, will always find her way to the room in the tower where she will touch the spindle as she tries to spin, unwittingly fulfilling the prophecy of the thirteenth wise woman. And who should hinder a youthful soul from climbing into the ancient tower and there beginning to spin? But when the soul awakens there in the head and feels its joy at seizing the threads of thought and spinning them further, it soon spins itself into its own little world. Quickly the soul is cocooned in a web of thoughts that cut it off from the realm of spirit which guided childhood existence. Under the tyranny of the head, doubt kills off a world of familiar fairy-tale figures and the whole palace falls under an evil spell.

But the princess in whom the whole firmament lives will not die. Twelve wise women stand by her cradle reflecting the powers of twelve constellations on to earth. "The princess shall not die but only fall into a deep hundred-year sleep," says the twelfth wise woman. For the being of the child is immortal; it can be enchanted but never destroyed. A hundred years is a long time, clever earth-reason will say; no-one could ever know that awakening will come after this explicit period of time. "World sleep" steals over the depths of the soul for a whole epoch while the intellect develops. But this epoch — the materialistic epoch — will one day pass away.

Even as a young person experiences the birth of reason with the coming of his earth maturity at puberty, thereby repeating mankind's experience, so he can also break through the magic spell of the intellect. Then the hundred years have passed for him. There were people graced by destiny to have this experience long ago, and they told beautiful fairy-tales of the awakening, for they themselves had met the Awakener who had kissed awake the eye of their soul and freed the palace from the magic spell. These people could say of the fairy-tale kings and princesses: "and though they have died yet one day will they arise again."

Indeed they can rise up again before an inward perception: Snow White and Cinderella, Tom Thumb and the poor miller's boy, the golden children and the little sister with the fawn. And they have lost nothing of their youthful freshness and sacred reality, for they are prototypes of our own soul's powers and stages of development. They are not allegories or symbols but real figures who have their own well-defined destinies and transformations. In all this there is more psychology than ordinary self-analysis can yield. But this soul reveals itself only to a vision which proceeds beyond sense-perception and sequential thinking to a direct experience of the formative powers in nature and in the life of the soul.

Rudolf Steiner described the attainment of this higher level of cognition from various angles. He called it "Imagination" because it leads into a realm of creative pictures. Our own inner life, which ordinarily comes before us only in memory pictures, moods and wishes, then expands to encompass an inner world of forms. The powers, light and dark, at work behind the individual impulses of the soul now take on the character of objects. When, by inner activity, thoughts begin to be transformed into Imagination, an inward experience occurs which renews the soul's life of feeling and perception; the individual feels younger as he grows into the imaginative world. The same formative forces which build up our bodies in childhood now instil a thinking built of creative pictures. Thus the soul's awakening is a return to earliest childhood. This sheds light on Christ's saying that we must first become as children before we may enter the kingdom of heaven.

There was a stage in human evolution when this picture-consciousness, a heritage of the heavens, was common to all. Then man did not seek the answer to riddles of knowledge in clear-cut concepts or through logical chains of thought, for the deeper interconnections were revealed to him in flowing pictures and life-filled figures. Man dreamed solutions to the secrets of the world. Today's dreaming, laced with the day's memories and steered by forces of desire, is only a poor remnant, a caricature of the old picture-vision which revealed itself all the more reliably the less reflective reasoning was involved.

It was instinctive wisdom which fashioned the great imaginations of the gods, creating the myths as picture-experiences with the certainty and exactitude of a natural force in man. Later this wisdom could still portray in sagas and legends the play of supersensory powers into human history. From it also arose the great symbolic pictures that accompany religious revelations and the symbolic language of ancient ritual.

Only with the progressive development of intellectual powers and the modern scientific attitude did those pristine faculties decline. They had to be sacrificed for the development of the free human personality, which required objective thinking. Above this present-day waking consciousness a new picture-experience can be developed: a "super-consciousness" which retains the clarity of pure thinking and has overcome desires and dream-life. While the fairy-tale is a remnant of ancient soul faculties which live on in a few people, it is also a prophetic forerunner leading towards the new picture-experience. It gives life to the power of imagination lightly dreaming beneath the intellectual layer of consciousness, powers which are already there pressing for development.

In *Heinrich von Ofterdingen,* Novalis depicts this imaginative power of the cognition which lies at the heart of genuine fairy-tales. He calls it "Fable".

"What seekest thou?" said the Sphinx.

"My own estate," replied Fable.

"Whence comest thou?"

"From olden times."

"Thou art yet a child."

"And shall be child eternally."
"Who will stand by thee in aid?"
"I stand for myself."

The fairy-tale is always seeking its own "estate" for in essence it always has to do with a return from exile, the self alienation of the human soul and the rediscovery of eternal childhood. But this childlikeness is not dim unconsciousness, it implies an intimate relationship with the world, the kind of knowledge that prevailed in earliest times. Because humanity must enter life through the gates of childhood, the fairy-tales will always be there. Their characters are woven from the light-filled substance of childhood which provides a fertile meeting point for the simplest young mind and the wisdom of age.

The brothers Jakob and Wilhelm Grimm did not assemble their collection of fairy-tales from a clear knowledge of their supersensory origin. But as true sons of Romanticism they had an innate feeling for the wisdom of the tales. They discerned the inner laws of the picture-sequences even though they could not grasp fully the nature of imaginative consciousness.

"Common to all fairy-tales," wrote Wilhelm Grimm, "is the residue of a belief which goes back to the most ancient times and speaks of supersensory things in picture-form. This mythical element resembles tiny fragments of a jewel, which lie scattered on the ground, overgrown with grass and flowers, evident only to a keenly discerning eye. Their significance has long been lost, but it can still be felt. This gives fairy-tales their content, and at the same time satisfies our natural pleasure in wonders. The fairy-tales are never a play of colours over empty fantasy."

Wilhelm Grimm never felt justified in making a pastiche of the motifs and developing them according to poetic fancy as did Arnim and Brentano. At the beginning of the nineteenth century it was still possible to gather these sacred fragments of folklore and preserve them intact without falsification by the intellect.

The brothers gathered the gems together from story-tellers in all areas. The pictures and words rose from the depths of their memory and they would not tolerate any altered phrase when the story was retold. The fairy-tale had a musical structure whose parts were woven into a unity. In later years Wilhelm developed the courage to fill in missing portions of the tales and felt more inclined to "tell them in his own way". This was the case for instance with "Snow White and Rose Red". But from this example it becomes obvious how carefully it was done. By constant immersion in the available fragments and meticulous attention to the laws which are implicit in the imaginations themselves, Wilhelm created versions that are far from spurious.

In the following observations we shall try to recover in the old folk-tales the lost significance of which Wilhelm Grimm speaks and the comprehension of the supersensory things through the images of Grimms' fairy-tales. Modern research has gathered a vast amount of material on fairy-tales and traced the connections of motifs among different races and cultures. While recognizing the diligence of this research, we are convinced that this method will never lead to real understanding of the fairy-tales. It does not trace the picture-motifs back to their original supersensory visionary source and in establishing the interdependence of fairy-tales it cannot conceive that related imaginations could be experienced by different peoples at different times. For although similar motifs often appear it is in the development of these motifs that the progress of human consciousness is revealed, and similar pictures in different contexts can express very different things. In imaginative experience the whole sequence of events is important, and the pictures should not be treated singly.

Perhaps the most important thing for our examination is to find, in each case, the inner starting point for the revelation of the supersensory: to discover the modes of consciousness out of which a particular imagination comes to expression. For that we need to feel our way into all that comprises the human being and his connection with the supersensory worlds. To discover such paths of spiritual striving is quite a different endeavour from an interpretation based on symbolism. This would destroy the stimulus of artistic experience and pleasure. Through the revelation of the spiritual sources the reader is encouraged to penetrate ever more deeply into the inner structure and pictures of the fairy-tale. Such an understanding will enhance our appreciation of the finer points which escape us if we regard the fairy-tale as no more than a brightly coloured play of fantasy.

It goes without saying that fairy-tales should be told to children without any explanation. The child unites himself quite naturally with the inner significance of the story. He absorbs the language of the imaginations and feels intimately related to it. The child's etheric formative forces, which determine the development and health of the body, are nourished by the fairy-tale pictures as though by an elixir of life. Fairy-tale wisdom is indeed ready to offer the "water of life" which today we all need to counterbalance hardening processes and death forces active in our organism from the earliest years.

If we make no attempt to gain conscious knowledge

of the spiritual sources from which the fairy-tale pictures arose, any sense for the higher reality which their characters express will soon be extinguished. Certainly it is a hopeful sign that the interest in folktales increases. But perhaps there is more to it than that. The heart knows more than the head will admit: the soul has a presentiment that the Awakener approaches to free it from enchantment.

2

The destiny of
primal wisdom

Fairy-tales are the deepest revelation of the folk mind and feeling. Nowhere does one meet the folk soul in its secret sufferings, victorious powers and purest longings so directly as in listening to its fairy-tales. It is as though a primal memory were the source of a stream which carries the motifs from generation to generation, as long as school dust has not covered the pure child-forces of the soul or the technology of civilization killed the feeling for imaginative pictures and their meaning. What then is this primal memory? We have already emphasized that it does not spring from the fable-making fantasy suggested by academics. It is not sufficient to see in all myths and fairy-tales merely an animistic "pagan" urge to ensoul nature. Jakob Grimm called it arrogant to suppose that the life of whole centuries was permeated with dull, unpleasant barbarity. "Paganism," he said, "never fell out of thin air. Untold ages were sustained by traditions derived originally from mysterious revelations which bore fruit in the wonderful language, creative faculties and the continued generation of mankind." The fairy-tale appears to us as the last shining afterglow of that "mysterious revelation" which must have stood at the beginning of all folk cultures, civilizations and customs — an inkling and a memory of the high origin of our human nature. The virgin human soul, which has to serve as Cinderella or Maid Maleen imprisoned in the dark tower, where neither sun nor moon shine in, is of royal descent. High up in a room in the tower sits Rapunzel, guarded by the witch. She would be cut off from the world like Maid Maleen, or sunk in the deep enchanted sleep like Brier Rose, if she no longer had her hair "as fine as spun gold". This golden hair she lets fall "twenty ells down" from the little window in the tower. To speak of golden hair is to portray ancient and holy powers of consciousness. A condition of illumination came over the soul from time to time: "Rapunzel, Rapunzel, let down your hair," calls the witch. Rapunzel has to comply for she is still under the spell of ancient atavistic powers. Such souls sank into a somnambulistic condition — "twenty ells down" — in which the waking consciousness was dimmed, to be replaced by a sunlike wisdom. The condition of rapture such as the Wala still experienced in Celtic and Germanic sanctuaries when spiritual vision was becoming rare, gives some idea of what is meant here. In the Greek world of sagas they spoke of the Golden Fleece (the ram's wool shining like the sun) which the Argonauts sought. But dark powers make use of these pure soul faculties. They rise from the depths, make the soul unfree, hold back its development. The witch, a fallen sibyl, appears as the bearer of regressive mediumistic abilities. The soul has to free itself from her spell by meeting its true self, the King's son, who climbs the golden streaming hair into the tower. But the path which leads from compulsion to the freedom of the individuality is hard. It demands first the renunciation of all shining wisdom: the soul must go through poverty and the wilderness before it can become a queen. Mercilessly the golden hair is shorn and Rapunzel cast out into loneliness.

In the "Goose Girl" the princess's path of suffering is told differently. Her mother gives her a maid to accompany and serve her on her travels. But the maid becomes arrogant and wishes to usurp the princess. The lower earthly personality, with its everyday thinking, a thinking that can easily puff itself up and posture as vastly knowledgeable, has become vainglorious; the maid has no mind to serve any more. The deeper intuition, the ancient original heritage of spirit, is mocked and dethroned where its inner nature is no longer understood.

What does it mean to feel these intuitive experiences arise? When the ancestors still spoke in the blood, when memories of past generations flashed up from the depths of the soul like memories of childhood days, then the soul became wise. Such people lived and acted out of an experience which extended far beyond the limits of their own lives. They were the bearers of a more comprehensive consciousness, for the blood in which the ancestral forces still worked on stored-up primal wisdom. This ancient heritage of spirit worked through the blood from generation to generation.

This inherited "blood" memory has gradually been expelled by our present day head-memory in the course of evolution. This process began when the tribes and families, which in ancient times led strictly self-contained lives, mixed their blood-line with strangers. Siegfried, who could understand the language of the birds, is a child of the marriage of brother and sister. The formative forces of the blood were then so rich that they could bear close marriages without deterioration. The transition from the near marriage to the far marriage, and finally to the mixing of nations, determine the point at which the intellect was born. At that point the instinctive forces of the soul had to fade away. From then on the personality, freed

21

from the narrow ties of kinship, could develop. The point of transition was of course earlier for some peoples and later for others but it always meant the darkening of the original wisdom and the fading of the old powers. That was the price paid for the awakening of individuality.

This necessity of evolution is often felt as a tragedy. The folk-soul, long abandoned by the divine powers, is depicted in the fairy-tales as a widow. The widow sends her daughter to a distant kingdom having promised her to a king's son. The individual soul, set free from the folk-soul must find the kingly power of the free individuality, achieved only by a long journey through strange lands.

In the ancient mystery schools the teacher spoke of the stage of homelessness which the disciple had to pass through before he was ready for the awakening of the eternal in his soul. We know that many of the wise men of antiquity were charged to travel; to become acquainted with foreign customs and ways of looking at things until in the course of time they acquired sufficient inner freedom. Only then was a wise man able to use his powers for the benefit of his own people; now he could give them laws from a higher wisdom, as did Solon to the Athenians after his travels. It is also told that Gautama Buddha stepped forth upon the way "from his home country into homelessness".

The tale of the "Goose Girl" seeks to evoke this mood of soul. It tells how the princess sets forth on her journey provided with rich treasures by her mother, the "widow". Before her daughter leaves, the old mother cuts her finger and lets three drops of blood fall on a white cloth. She gives this to her daughter, saying: "Take good care of this. You will need it on your journey". For as Goethe said, "blood is a very special fluid"; whoever possesses it is master of the human being concerned. Both angels and demons fight for the blood through which the striving individuality can unfold its activity. The princess mounts her talking horse Fallada, and leaves with her maid. Becoming thirsty she asks her maid to bring her water in her golden goblet. The maid refuses so the princess dismounts to drink. The incident is repeated and the princess inadvertently drops the white cloth into the stream. The maid finds it and now has power over the princess, who without the drops of blood becomes weak and helpless. The maid orders the princess to change clothes with her and hand over her horse.

As long as the soul retains in the blood its connection with the holiest forces of its people, the resonance of inspired consciousness can still work on. Only when the princess loses the drops of her mother's blood does her pristine knowledge vanish. She has to surrender Fallada to the maid, who promptly announces herself as the bride when they reach the court of a foreign king. The maid has Fallada's head cut off fearing that the horse will give away her secret; but at the request of the princess, now a goose girl, the head is nailed to the wall of the town's gateway.

In old Germanic cultures, the horse was treated with religious reverence. The love which bound gods and heroes to their horses is well known. The horse appears in sagas and myths as a picture of the instinctive forces of the understanding. When it appears as a winged steed — like Pegasus — it is seen as the imagination: the flight of thought which is able to free itself from the heaviness of earth and fly up to the super-terrestrial. In the Four Horseman of the Apocalypse we find reflected consecutive stages in the development of human intelligence: from white to red, and then to the black and the pale horse. At the end of time the white horseman returns from on high and founds a new kingdom in which the spirit is victorious. At the very beginning of mankind's striving, the light-filled forces of wisdom are still present. The wise instincts are caught by the desire-nature (red) and finally darken to the earthbound intellect, which only measures and counts (black). And in materialism they are misused more and more by the destructive forces: death rides upon the pale horse. The direction of the will, active in thinking, is always the decisive factor: this is revealed in the form and colour of the horse. Only the future will bring the triumph of the light-filled heavenly wisdom over a thinking that is in decline. Then the white horseman will appear in a new form in the earthly realm.

The "Goose Girl" depicts the fading of the ancient wisdom in the soul. The earth-consciousness has become arrogant, knows only low cunning, and is no longer willing to serve. It has been given to the soul as servant on the path of human evolution. But it dethrones the girl, kills the inspiring powers of wisdom, and takes full possession of the personality. The maid marries the king's son and the princess looks after the geese. It is a telling picture of a particular attitude of soul. The senses are similar to a flock of geese, forever running after the attractions of the surrounding world and constantly in danger of losing themselves in sensations. There is a stage on the way to the spirit — and this is especially characteristic of the Western way — which can be described thus: the princess becomes a goose girl. The soul must learn to tend the senses carefully but must not suppress or deaden them. For a false asceticism would lead only to a stunting of the inner nature of the human being rather than development of the hidden spiritual powers. The soul must learn to travel through the earthly world with the senses awake but under its sovereign rule.

The soul that strengthens itself in this way learns to experience the moments of waking up and falling asleep in a particular way: a primal consciousness glimmers in the depths and a long-dead knowledge begins to speak. In the fairy-tale the Goose Girl walks through the dark gateway every morning and evening with her flock of geese and talks with the horse's head: "Oh, poor Fallada, hanging there," and the horse replies: "Oh, poor princess in despair, if your dear mother knew, her heart would break in two." The seeds of higher consciousness lie in these moments between waking and sleeping. Gradually, out of confused dream-pictures, echoes of the day's experiences, more significant pictures emerge and out of the dimness of sleep shines the memory of a far-off kingdom. The soul remembers her royal descent. Painfully it recalls all that has been lost.

The Goose Girl out in the meadow combs her golden hair and it glistens in the sunshine. She catches the flowing light of wisdom: the rays of the sun begin to think within her. However she has to learn to order and nurture this streaming light. It is the way of immersion and self-observation which is portrayed in such pictures. There is also a nice humorous touch — for without some sovereign humour it is impossible to find the true spirit — when cheeky Conrad wants to pull the princess's hair as she combs it out, and she calls up the wind to blow the boy away. We all have a Conrad living in us. He likes to inject his impertinent sense of fun into the calmness of reflective thinking and does not allow devotion and reverence to arise. Anyone who wishes to immerse himself in the sources of wisdom must learn to send away the flickering play of whimsical notions. How can that be done?

The original wisdom of the Nordic peoples was cast in alliterative rhymes and powerfully magic rhythms. Odin, who reigns in the breath, was the master of rune-magic. He was the god of the skalds and taught them to send the holy power of speech into the breath. The skald felt himself to be the steward of the might of words; the noblest powers of the gods were entrusted to him when he shaped his words. And so he said that he had been appointed master of the wind. Thus, in the experience of speech, the soul comprehended the continuing creative activity of the spirit, for world-will still operated in the revelation of speech. He who had learned to comprehend the world spirit in the word (in the rune) raised himself above the pale, deceptive thinking of the intellect. The power of language, cast into rhythm and alliteration, carried the soul far above itself, uniting it with the creative breath of world-wisdom. The fairy-tale refers to this mighty experience. The princess is able to cast a spell upon the wind for she has influence over the breath through the word filled with the power of the gods. Where holy singing sounds, where the rune-wisdom of the skalds resounds, Conrad has no power. It is the magic of poetry which can chase away the intellect which pulls everything to pieces.

Finally the King becomes suspicious and questions the Goose Girl. On his advice she confides her plight to the iron stove, for she had sworn to the maid never to tell anyone what had happened to her. While the princess climbs into the stove and bewails her fate the king stands outside and overhears her confession. Here, the fairy-tale touches on a mystery of the heart. A picture of a stove, particularly a red-hot fiery stove, often plays a part in dreams. It is not difficult to see that an excitement of the heart or a feverish condition of the body can be reflected by such a symbol. Another of Grimms' fairy-tales, the "Cast-iron Stove", tells of a king's son sitting in a cast-iron stove, under a spell, waiting for the princess who can release him. Here we are told of the liberation of royal spirit-powers held prisoner by the petrification of the heart. In the "Goose Girl", the opposite happens: the princess must go into the stove. In order that the spiritual experience can become effective the soul must learn to go down to the deepest depths of the heart. The heart must be able to transform the supersensory wisdom the spirit has attained into a fully human experience. In the last resort it is impossible for the earthly intellect to give expression to the soul's memory of its true origin and the realization of its mission. To fully perceive oneself as an eternal being is an action of the deepest holiness: it cannot be communicated from person to person. It is a mystical fact which involves a secret act of self-awakening. The soul must acknowledge afresh its descent and origin. The picture of the old king listening from his hiding-place as the Goose Girl speaks the secret of her destiny, portrays the ancient spirit-consciousness that stands unseen behind our musings and strivings. This is the power which forms our destinies. Hitherto it has led and commanded us, but it can declare that we have come of age. This guiding power — the old king — understands what the heart speaks to itself and, thus, can judge and rescue.

The human soul has to undergo poverty on the path that leads to inner freedom. When ancient wisdom was extinguished in the blood, the earthly intellectual consciousness began to dominate and rob the soul of its royal dignity. The eternal heritage of the spirit is threatened with extinction as it passes through the world of the senses. The lower personality suppresses the memory of the soul's true origin. But in this journey ordained by destiny, the soul is thrown back upon itself in order to develop an inner freedom which, by a powerful act of self-recollection, leads it back to the spirit. Then the soul can celebrate its "royal wedding".

3

Snippets of knowledge

The fading of the fairy-tale characters from our lives is the work of a very clever deceiver who appears in numerous stories in the guise of the tailor. He is the arrogant intellect which cuts everything to pieces with learned and detailed explanations in order to sew it together again in a different way.

The fairy-tale has its own way of stating its case. It simply describes someone who can do nothing but measure and analyse as a stay-at-home: a dried-up tailor busy with scissors, needle and thread. From the fairy-tale viewpoint it is important to imagine how such a tailor would behave in heaven. When the human intellect, in its presumption, pits itself against the divine mysteries, something grotesque appears in the cosmos. The intellect has no idea how absurd it looks when it tries to unravel the riddles of existence with its mundane ideas.

Fortunately humour comes to the rescue. The "Tailor in Heaven" shows the tailor arriving at heaven's gate after a long and tiring journey. But the Lord and all the apostles and saints have gone out for a stroll in the heavenly garden. Only Peter is left and he has instructions to admit no one during the Lord's absence.

It is important to pay attention to dates indicated in such fairy-tales for they provide a key to understanding the spiritual situation. Here it clearly points to a post-Christian stage in human evolution. The apostles and saints are certainly there, but they are not enthroned in heaven or taking part in earthly events. In fact, the heavenly retinue is, so to speak, not at home. Only Peter remains as custodian and he has the duty of seeing that no one should peer into heaven. Clearly the times described are those when mankind had to acquiesce to tradition and dogma. One can understand this as a necessity in human evolution by observing how the capacity of thinking began to develop when the answers to questions no longer came by grace. The urge to philosophize and to solve the riddles of existence by one's own power could evolve only when the gods withdrew and the heavens remained closed.

Human thinking sets out to conquer the heavens. It knocks at heaven's door and it is remarkable how the "honest little tailor" as he styles himself, is greeted by Peter. "As honest as a thief on the gallows," says Peter. "You've been light-fingered, you've filched snippets of cloth." But the tailor will not be turned away. "Have mercy," he pleads. "It's not stealing to take wee little scraps that fall off the table all by themselves." Here we touch on something axiomatic, for a tailor — in heaven's eyes — cannot be other than "light-fingered". Rudolf Steiner describes how human head-nature (sense-observation and thinking) in contra-distinction to the limb-nature, always has a "kleptomanic" attitude to the world. It is quite justifiable, for example, if a young person eager to learn and thirsty for knowledge adopts ideas discovered by others. The head-nature recognizes no mine or thine. But when this attitude rightly assumed by the head shifts to the limbs the illness of kleptomania arises. If the head-forces develop one-sidedly and extend into the feeling and will nature, this illness can appear as a temporary disturbance of the maturing being. In the earthly realm the intellect with its greed for knowledge is a kleptomaniac, and necessarily so. But once it approaches the threshold of the spiritual world it must become aware of this attitude of mind. What exists of right in the realm of the senses is harmful in supersensory realms and must be laid aside for there only wisdom bought with the heart's blood is valid. The light of knowledge which is not ensouled with the warmth of experience has no illuminating power in the higher worlds.

In Goethe's fairy-tale, of the "Green Snake and the Beautiful Lily", the tailor motif appears in the guise of two will o' the wisps. Instead of "sticky fingers", they have long tongues and they lick the gold from everything they find. But they cannot retain it and shed it at every suitable and unsuitable opportunity. Many who eat it die, but the Green Snake can digest and absorb it and become inwardly illumined. The snake, transformed and transfigured by the gold, is ready to sacrifice herself. She builds the bridge over the river and prepares the way to the other realm, which the will o' the wisps can never enter. The person who can only turn wisdom into ideas, without translating it into inner activity and experiencing its transforming power, remains a poor wight. In the face of spiritual realities, his striving for knowledge avails him nothing.*

In the "Tailor in Heaven", Peter, out of pity, lets the tailor into heaven on the condition that he will sit meekly in a corner behind the door. The tailor, however, is curious and goes prowling about looking into every corner. He finds the golden seat where the

* See Rudolf Steiner's "The Character of Goethe's Spirit" in Goethe, *The Fairy Tale*, Steiner Publications, New York, and Floris Books, Edinburgh, 1979.

Lord sits and rules the earth. Of course the tailor cannot restrain himself from sitting on the golden seat, where he can see everything happening on earth. He sees a washerwoman stealing and, since everyone has least patience with those failings to which they are most prone, is very indignant, hurling a golden footstool at the thief. Returning, the Lord discovers the missing stool. The tailor has to confess. "You scoundrel!" says the Lord. "If I were to judge like you, what do you suppose would have happened to *you* long ago? And besides, all my chairs, benches, tables, even my fire tongs would be gone; I'd have thrown them all at sinners." The tailor is turned out of heaven for, "There's only one judge here in heaven, and that's me, the Lord."

The judging intellect fails in moderation. It wants to see at work in the sphere of justice the same laws that are connected with cause and effect in the realm of nature. But if the moral order of the world allowed expiation to follow hard on guilt, the earthly world would have been utterly destroyed long ago. Human deeds and destined atonement are not visibly connected. They are often separated by great spaces of time for cosmic justice wisely interweaves the outcome of human deeds into the progressive development of the human race. The tailor who seats himself on the Lord's throne and hurls a footstool at a sinner is not unlike the theology which, in its zeal to champion the honour of God, hastens to condemn. It lacks knowledge of the great rhythms of evolution. The laws of destiny begin to disclose themselves only to one who has overcome impatience and can trust in the stream of time. Earthly powers of judgment, especially moral judgments, create forces of disturbance in the higher worlds.

There is another side to the tailor for he can fight with
the giants, bid for the hand of a royal princess and
become ruler of a great kingdom. In these images we
see musty and outworn powers succumbing to the
forces of thinking. The bearers of atavistic instinctive
powers must give way to the clear intellectual consciousness. This, at first, seems powerless and
unhallowed in comparison with the ancient gifts which
once enriched the soul. The early mode of consciousness though, in which the human soul would bask as if
spread out over the whole world, gigantically but
dreamily, has been long on the wane. A mere ghost of
it casts its shadow upon the soul here and there. It is
the giant's shadow in Goethe's fairy-tale which the will
o' the wisps can use at twilight to reach the other shore
of existence. But wherever the clear light of knowledge rules, the power of the giant fades away.

In the "Brave Little Tailor", the keenly awake
intelligence makes itself lord over the giants. The
tailor's secret of success is self-confidence. He knows
how to bluff: "What a man am I?" he says, admiring his
own cleverness. "The whole town must hear of this."
And the little tailor cuts a belt and stitches on it in large
letters, "Seven at one blow!" That the seven were
merely flies need not be immediately admitted to the
world.

All intellectual knowledge has an inherent urge to
make itself widely known. Scholars want to gain
recognition for their ideas, inventors to put their
inventions to use, the "enlightened" to change the
world. They cannot wait. "Town, my foot! The whole
world must hear of it!" says the tailor, and he dons his
belt and swaggers out into the world, for of course his
workshop is too small for his cleverness. Belief in the
power of the intellect alone to enhance life makes short
shrift of tradition and custom. Ancient forms totter

and fall, surrendering to the intellect without testing what is so confidently applauded. A swindler's sorcery is behind the behaviour of the little tailor, as the fairy-tale shows very clearly. It portrays how the world can be taken by storm. Yet one can see that the tailor has his mission for he acts in the spirit of the times when he sets out to put old powers in their place.

The "Giant and the Tailor" tells how a tailor takes service with a giant — a significant touch. When the tailor asks what wage he will be paid, the giant answers: "Every year you shall have 365 days, with an extra day in leap year. What do you say to that?" The primal depths of our consciousness are powerless during the day when earthly thinking and sense impressions dominate. But this earthly intellect is presumptuous; it has not yet become conscious of its limitations and thinks it can comprehend the world in its totality. The tailor forgets that he lives by the favour of the giant: were he not active ever renewing the body out of cosmic wisdom during sleep, the tailor would not have the 365 days of the year.

But it is quite another story when the "Clever Little Tailor"hears of the proud princess who sets all her suitors riddles then dismisses them with a scornful laugh. Fairy-tale princesses know that a happy marriage depends on whether the man is good at learning from riddles. Three tailors appear before the princess and she asks her riddle: "I have two kinds of hair on my head. What colours are they?"

"Nothing to it," says the first tailor, "they must be black and white like the cloth called pepper-and-salt." Of course he has guessed wrong for his concepts are bound to the commonplace. He thinks no further than the stuff which occupies him all day long.

The second tailor soars a bit higher. "If it's not black and white," he says, "it's brown and red like my father's frock coat." This tailor loves the festive moments of life, even though it may only be the family feasts for which his father's dinner jacket is brought out of the cupboard. His conceptual powers fall short of approaching a princess's secret.

Only the third tailor achieves the solution for he speaks of gold and silver, and these are not colours a tailor deals with in his workshop. Gold and silver indicate the cosmos. The sun's radiance and the moon's glimmer live in the thoughts of the youngest tailor for his imagination has the power to soar and apprehend the super-earthly. For the princess — and that is indeed her riddle — is "not of this world". Whoever would join his fate with hers must first awaken in his own soul something which is of heavenly rather than earthly origin.

But it takes more than that to raise oneself on the wings of the soul to the super-earthly and thus unite the heavenly with one's earthly existence so that it imbues the transitory personality with the nature of the eternal and imperishable. No tailor becomes a king's son so quickly: he must first prove himself. The princess commands him to spend the night with a bear.

In fairy-tale philosophy we constantly encounter the deep connection between man and beast — not in the Darwinian sense but from an understanding that animals are beings who have not yet reached the goal of human existence. They have remained behind and sigh for the "glorious liberty" of the children of God! This is the longing of the whole creation, which, being subject to transience, looks to redeemed humanity for help. The truly wise have always perceived this, as Paul described in his Epistle to the Romans. The bear — think of the bewitched, good- natured bear in "Snow White and Rose Red" — is a transformed sense-picture of this longing of the creature to become human.

Anyone who has seen a performing bear standing on its hind legs can detect something of this urge of the creature to reach beyond itself and also of the weight of gravity which draws it down again to its earth-bound posture. Anyone who has seen this has gained some idea of what bewitchment is. Many things are still bewitched and earth-bound within ourselves. Every night, when we sleep, we pay tribute to the earthly laws ruling our limbs. And whoever dreams of the gold and silver hair of a princess and can soar to the heavens, must ever again remember that he is not only spirit but body also. Otherwise everything that obeys earth's gravity will one day rise against the visionary and draw him down, all the more deeply, into its realm.

The tailor who has solved the riddle must show that he knows how to get on with the bear. The clever little tailor does not fight the bear for he knows how to hold its brute strength in check without slaying it. For this, one needs humour and a gift for being continually watchful and resourceful. He tries to hold the active interest of his dumb companion, first by cracking nuts for he who can guess the riddles knows how to crack nuts. But instead of nuts the bear is given stones which he vainly tries to crack. The stupid senses are greedy for knowledge but submissive when they begin to realize that faculties other than brute force exist. Now the tailor takes his violin and plays a tune. The bear begins to dance for music releases him from the power of gravity. Soon he wants to play the violin and begs the tailor to teach him. The tailor incapacitates the bear by fastening his paws on the pretext of cutting his nails so he can play the violin. By showing that he knows how to control the bear the tailor has proved his royal worth. The spirit has overcome earthly gravity.

When Socrates was dying, he spoke of his "daimon", his good genius who was always reminding him:

"Socrates, practise music!" He took it to mean that he should bravely continue to philosophize, for was not philosophy also a gift of the muses? But his genius really meant music: a life of rhythm and artistic sense-activity. Socrates is the forefather of those who experience their highest joy in dismembering ideas and putting them together again: an honest-to-goodness tailor! The full reality of earth threatened to pass him by. He wanted to lead the Greeks from the fullness of their sense-life to regions of the spirit for the body seemed to him but the prison of the soul. The Greeks instinctively rebelled against this.

The tailor must take a violin with him to master the bear. At that moment the heavy earth-force will be raised to the spirit; otherwise it will revenge itself on anyone who despises the sense-nature.

4

Helpful beings

In the fairy-tale world belief in the good powers and their wise guidance prevails. Man is never abandoned to poverty or oppression. The wisdom of destiny usually works in a wonderful progression of events and needs no particular being through which to reveal itself. However, sometimes a wise counsellor is introduced, who sets tasks and exacts conditions.

In the "Water of Life" the counsellor takes the guise of an old man who advises three princes how to save their ailing father. In the "Shoes that were Danced Through" an old woman explains to a soldier the mystery of how the twelve princesses, night after night, wear out their shoes. "Just don't drink the wine they bring you in the evening, and then pretend to be fast asleep." She gives him a cloak and tells him: "When you put this on, you will be invisible and you'll be able to follow the twelve princesses."

In such counsel it is not difficult to recognize that the answer to the question of how to remain conscious when falling asleep, in order to watch the mysterious processes of sleep, is to refrain from the intoxicating drink offered up from the forces of the bodily nature. The soul must understand the stupefying effects of the fumes streaming up to the head on falling asleep. Here the soldier (the man already established in life) is set apart. While he has acquired a certain life experience, he now has to learn to awaken free of the physical body on a higher level and move in the region of the soul in supersensory spirit-form: that is, to receive the cloak of invisibility.

Other helpers do their work for mankind in hidden ways. After "Snow White and Rose Red" have spent the night sleeping in a wood, they see a beautiful child in a shining white garment sitting near them. It is the angel who has watched by the precipice on the edge of which they had unwittingly fallen asleep.

In "Mary's Child", the Virgin Mary takes the three-year-old child into her own realm. At the age of three the child awakens to its consciousness of self and needs forces other than inheritance to nourish its soul-life. Spiritual forces of motherhood must now watch over its growth. They must, so to speak, lay the blue mantle of the Madonna over the forces quickening in the soul so that the faculties of thinking, feeling and willing unfold correctly. Attitudes of reverence and wonder should be especially cultivated in a child's heart at this time. Everything that nourishes the soul of the growing child with pictures that teach one to apprehend the divine, originates in the wise cherishing care of the heavenly mother. At fourteen the young soul grows beyond these bounds, breaking through the protective shell in which it has been sheltered. It becomes conscious of its earthly body and independence: Mary's child falls out of the heavens and finds herself living in a hollow tree.

Other helpers again are the "fairies" which mediate between the circles of heaven and the earth and endow the child in the cradle with their gifts. The human being receives its form and disposition of soul from the twelve regions of the zodiac. Twelve fairies bestow them. Brier-Rose begins life richly endowed, for she is a heavenly plant. But most often, the fairy-tales tell of the helpful power of the elementals. The dwarves who search in the hills for ore, and the gnomes active in the realm of roots and crystal, have little difficulty finding a connection with the seeking human soul. They bear a clear intelligence which penetrates nature's laws without strained thinking, and regard the human being as a thick-head. So they strive to enlighten man and remind us to be aware and awake. Through listening to the hidden forces active around us and participating with love in the world, the higher organs of the soul are awakened. But often intellectual pride hinders the soul from following the advice of the gnomes.

In the "Water of Life", the eldest prince, who sets off to seek the restorative potion, meets a dwarf on the road. "Where are you going so fast?" the dwarf asks. "You stupid runt," replies the prince haughtily, "what business is it of yours?" This makes the little man furious and he sets a curse upon him. It is not too long before the prince rides into a ravine where he can neither turn his horse around nor dismount. Logical thinking which shuts itself off from fructifying forces of natural phenomena, ends up going nowhere.

The second brother meets the same fate, but the third stops to talk to the dwarf and is told: "Since you have spoken kindly and haven't been haughty like your two brothers, I'll tell you where the Water of Life is and how to get there. It springs from the fountain in the courtyard of an enchanted castle, but you'll never get in unless I give you an iron wand and two loaves of bread. Strike the castle gate three times with the wand and it will open. Inside, there will be two lions with gaping jaws, but if you throw a loaf to each of them, they will calm down. Then you must hurry and take the Water of Life before the clock strikes twelve, because otherwise the gate will be closed and you will be locked in." The supersensory world does not lie wide open to the soul's gaze. One must possess active forces to open the door. The soul itself has to learn to be firm in the spirit and to be strong as it awakens: the fairy-tale tells us that an iron rod is needed to beat on the door if we would open it. When the soul enters the "castle" and presses forward to observe its own inner world, it encounters the powers unleashed from its own depths. The will-nature would overcome and bewilder the consciousness if the soul did not produce strong powers of thought. As the fairy-tale says: loaves of bread must be taken to pacify the lions.

The prince finds the Water of Life shortly before midnight and manages to carry it to safety before the clock strikes. Indeed whenever we fall into deep sleep we drink of this spring and receive new life from its waters which counteract the dying tendency of daytime existence on our organism. The sacred sources of life are at our disposal if we have knowledge of them. Initiation into this wisdom of healing can be attained during sleep, but not in the condition of deep sleep: the prince must leave before midnight.

The two elder princes do not seek the well of life in a selfless way, hoping to win their father's kingdom for themselves. Self-seeking is a force that narrows the soul and imprisons the searching princes in the ravine in the mountains. A true seeker of the spirit must radiate a love which will open the spiritual worlds to him. The attitude of the third brother is seen in his unwillingness to return to his father without his brothers. "Dear Dwarf, could you tell me where my two brothers are?" he asks. But the dwarf warns him: "Don't trust them. They have wicked hearts." And indeed, although they owe their freedom to the intercession of the third brother, they proceed to destroy the fruit of all toil. It is only after great pains that the good brother receives his dues, while the other two are punished.

The faculty of love is a necessity for the soul that aspires to penetrate knowledgeably into life's mysteries. And to bring supersensory wisdom actively into earthly existence, vigilance and judgment are needed. If what is sacred is to be preserved the ability to judge between the true and the false must be healthily developed.

The tale of the "Three Little Men in the Woods" also shows how a relationship between the human soul and the elemental beings can be established. The nature spirits become mediators for the holy life-forces which they wish to reveal to human beings. The story, a winter mystery, tells of a pious girl whose hard-hearted stepmother orders her to gather strawberries in the snow-covered forest. A love of the impossible is in the true fairy-tale vein. Into this wintry cold the child, clad only in a thin paper dress, is thrust with only a dry crust of bread to eat. She comes to the house in the forest where three dwarves live and shyly taps at the door.

Fairy-tales depict the mood of soul felt by seekers of the spirit when entering the elemental world as a feeling of loneliness; of standing entirely on one's own feet. So man, when no longer surrounded and cherished by human sympathy and warmth of feeling, must call upon his own warmth and heart forces, revealing in his progress on the lonely spirit-path how rich the sources of love which arise from the depths of the soul are.

The human soul is appointed to carry the purest powers of love into the spiritual worlds and it is for this that many elemental beings hunger. Sympathy is for them a nourishing and animating force. The girl has to prove she is ready to give her bread to the little men. When she gives them half of it, they ask her what she wants. The dwarves tell her to sweep away the snow behind the house, where she discovers the dark-red strawberries. In such pictures a Christmas mystery can be discerned. When we wish to experience rightly the birth of Christ we have "to brush away the snow" and bring to light the hidden mystery of life: the warmth of love which emerges from the cold of the world.

The red strawberries reveal the forces related to the blood-system which is also an effective means of healing. In pictures such as this we see the descent of the Christ-force into the crystalline clarity of thought. The sun-warmth of the Christ-love seeks to illuminate the wintry cold of the intellect. The fairy-tale shows how a relationship with the helpful nature spirits who rule over this Christmas mystery can shed blessings on the human soul. While the girl sweeps the snow away and gathers the strawberries, the little men decide to reward her. One promises that she shall become more beautiful day by day; the second, that gold shall fall from her lips whenever she speaks; and the third, that a king shall take her as his bride.

Finding the Christ-activity in the wintry world radiates into the formative life-forces of the human being. The Christ-force begins to spiritualize the human form and a new beauty, expressing itself from within, is granted to such a person. He who lives in touch with the good powers and shares in their activity may imbue his words with a higher reality: his speech enriches its hearers. Finally, the soul which occupies itself with the Christmas mystery finds its higher self. It can allow the royal powers of the spirit to penetrate it more and more deeply: a king comes and unites himself with the girl.

The idle girl on the other hand, although carefully clothed by her mother in furs and well supplied with food, searches the forest in vain. She finds no strawberries for she refuses to share her food with the three dwarves nor will she sweep away the snow. So the winter mystery passes her by. Her heart is insensitive to the warmth of love which can release life from the crystal cold. She is judged by the nature spirits and becomes uglier day by day for her soul is not penetrated by spirit. Whenever she speaks a toad falls from her mouth, for the coldness of her soul is in her speech and she sheds antipathy around her; finally she dies an unhappy death, for she has used only the death-forces in her soul during earth existence.

In these pictures we see the judgment of destiny acting through the wisdom-filled activities of the nature spirits. Through them the morality and the immorality of our aims and deeds is shaped into natural forces, which reveal themselves in our physical appearance, our gifts or our weaknesses.

The nature spirits work in the sprouting, blossoming and fruit-bearing realm of plants. An understanding of their working and weaving can, through anthroposophy, be raised to clear knowledge. Rudolf Steiner has shown that through imaginative knowledge we can experience the four elements — earth, water, air and fire — in a new way. In all activity that tends towards solidity, the gnomes (or dwarves) reveal themselves; in all that flows, the undines; the sylphs in the wafted scents and colours shining in the air; and salamanders in the fire-processes. These elemental beings weave their fourfold dance in the coming-into-being and the passing-away of the plants — in the cycle of root, leaf, blossom and seed-formation.

We admire the miracle of plant-growth, the blossoming tree or the ripening corn, while our senses are aware of them. But at night, when our souls pass into the surrounding worlds, our sense of wonder is transformed. Our soul feels worthless and inadequate when we become aware of how, for example, a cornfield ripens, and the miracle of a mysterious alchemy that charms the golden corn out of the bare blade. The elemental spirits can in reality spin straw into gold! They can accomplish more than the human being, in spite of his skills and technical knowledge. The soul, however proud of human progress it may be during the day, is overwhelmed at night by this wisdom-filled art. It feels worthless, tormented, and paralysed and this mood often remains during the day. These experiences have a lasting effect, even when in our waking hours we no longer remember them. "You pride yourself on being so wise and clever," an inner voice whispers, "but if you cannot spin straw into gold in our world you are nothing."

Riddles of knowledge can become deep problems of existence. At the threshold of the spiritual world they become trials of the soul, in which it is a question of "to be or not to be" when faced with supersensory beings. In "Rumpelstiltskin" the king tells the miller's daughter: "Now, get to work. You have the whole night ahead of you, but if you haven't spun this straw into gold by tomorrow morning, you will die."

Goethe represents Faust in his monologue as driven by thirst for knowledge, and breaking through the bounds of the supersensory world. Faust "conjures up the Earth Spirit": he becomes aware of the weaving and working of the elemental beings, but without being ripe for such knowledge. Man can recognize in the spirit only what he can in a certain sense become. He must learn to transmute himself into the nature of the higher worlds otherwise he will be turned back from them.

Rudolf Steiner describes why life in the sense-world is a necessity for the soul. It must here "develop a consciousness ... which in a certain respect lives in fixed ideas, vigorously forced upon it." Thus it will become so firmly established within itself that, later, in supersensory worlds of fleeting pictures and continual transformations it can maintain itself in full independence. This is the power which Faust has not fully developed. He is turned back from the threshold of the spiritual world and falls under the influence of a supersensory being whose true nature he cannot penetrate and from whom he cannot release himself. There, it is Mephistopheles; in "Rumpelstiltskin" it is an elemental spirit who offers his services, but in return possesses the human soul.

"If the soul is too weak for conscious experience in the elemental world," Rudolf Steiner writes, "its independence vanishes on entering there, just as a thought does which is not imprinted with sufficient clearness on the soul to live on as a distinct memory. In this case the soul cannot really enter the supersensory world at all with its consciousness ... And even if the soul has, so to speak, nibbled at the supersensory world so that, on sinking back into the physical world it retains something of the supersensory in its consciousness, such spoil from another sphere often only causes confusion in the life of thought."*

The ability to set thoughts in logical order is easily lost by people who have irregularly "nibbled" at the supersensory. Rumpelstiltskin demands the necklace from the miller's daughter: the power of experiencing oneself continuously as an independent personality finally disappears for this depends on the power of memory we have developed within the sense-world. Rumpelstiltskin also demands her ring. A ring is a sign that one belongs to someone else: it binds the

* *Die Schwelle der geistigen Welt.* (1913). (GA 17) Dornach 1972.

consciousness to a pledge. If, in a fairy-tale, a ring is lost or received one has to ask what the soul was formerly united with or what forces it is making a new connection with. Man can enter into pacts and undertake obligations by virtue of his spirit-nature. It raises him as a spiritual being above the rest of creation which can only be "possessed" and succumbs therefore to "enchantment". The true self can practise loyalty: it knows the secret of the ring. It follows that the soul, which more and more abandons control over itself, cannot reap the fruit of its intercourse with supersensory worlds. The new life which proceeds from union with the royal powers of the spirit falls apart or is forfeited to the demonic being who has gained the upper hand: Rumpelstiltskin demands the first child the miller's daughter shall bear the king.

To free oneself from the influence of such an elemental spirit one must recognize it for what it really is. He who fails to recognize the elementals, their power and their attributes, is no master of the spirits, cries Faust, as he conjures up the four elemental spirits by name. To know a being's name means to know its secret. To confront the hobgoblin Rumpelstiltskin with his name breaks the spell. In anthroposophical terminology Rumpelstiltskin is an Ahrimanic being, for he reveals his true nature in an outbreak of anger. He does not want to be recognized working most effectively in the depths of human nature where the light of consciousness does not usually penetrate. Because he lives as a parasite on the soul's powers, he gradually distorts the healthy working of the personality. Rumpelstiltskin represents a certain kind of darkening of the consciousness and its inevitable decline. In order to free oneself from such demonic powers one must recognize that it is a question of "possession". The elemental powers which are at work wisely and healthily in external nature become demonic as soon as they invade human nature and begin to rise up out of the realm of desire. Coming into contact with the world of supersensory powers in the wrong way, which can happen quite subconsciously, is often the deeper cause of such illnesses.

Fairy-tale wisdom describes the manifold interest taken by the nature-spirits in human evolution. The seven dwarves across the seven mountains, to whom Snow White comes when she is seven years old, are movingly described as kind beings, with a childlike nature. By the seventh year the child's body has been transformed from the inherited form to a physiognomy and posture expressing the personality of the individual. Losing the milk-teeth is a sign of this process. This personal bodily form or gestalt, which has at least partially overcome the inherited forces, is like the snow that falls from the heavens, having descended and been formed from the invisible worlds in virgin purity. One can find no more suitable name for it than Snow White.

In a hidden manner the human spirit is continuously creative. Everything fashioned by this essence — expressions and bodily gestures — radiates during sleep into the life-forces of nature. Rudolf Steiner describes how, to imaginative contemplation, a human spirit appears more gleaming and radiant when it brings to expression in countenance or gesture the wealth of its inner life. Gnomes and undines are aware of this creative spirit and admire its beauty. But until the child's seventh year, this creative power can barely come to expression. It remains invisible for the elementals for it is still living in the inherited body. Rudolf Steiner describes how those beings marvel that at a certain time the human form appears. They are full of curiosity and long to experience what this child had lived through before it became "visible". One cannot give them more delight than by telling them of childhood. They accept this with great gratitude and in return inspire the human soul with fairy-tale images. Out of this dialogue between human beings and nature spirits the fairy-tale mood is born. The conversations with nature spirits can be so gentle and fleeting that people are not always quite conscious of them. Only the fairy-tale mood remains and out of this mood the images well up: images and pictures which bear their own legitimacy. And because human hearts are alike the world over, similar motifs and images often appear. But one must not jump to the conclusion that this always indicates an interdependence. It would be interesting to trace the wanderings of related fairy-tale forms through different races and geological conditions. One would discover a variety of dispositions amongst the different kinds of elemental beings, each revealing in the temperament of their narratives their own peculiar kind of inspiration.

The human being, a riddle and a marvel, is greeted with astonishment in the realm of the nature spirits: that is the primal experience of the fairy-tale imagination. In the seventh year this being becomes visible. When Snow White was seven years old "she was as beautiful as the day," relates the fairy-tale. But her proud stepmother could not bear this. The vain earth-consciousness, which so loves to look in the mirror and gets its nourishment from its own reflection, has no sense for the divinely beautiful figure which, from its seventh year, longs to work through the hard shell of its body. From now on this spirit form of the human being, made up of heavenly forces, lights up in the elemental regions. The dwarves discover her in their realm and greet the sleeping child with admiration.

From this time of life onwards the soul begins a mysterious dialogue with the elemental beings. They need each other, for the human soul is, so to speak, brought up by the elementals. The gnomes gladly help Snow White to become aware of herself. But the tragedy is that they cannot protect her from the stupefying and poisonous influences of the sense nature. Snow White succumbs to the wicked step-mother because she is not sufficiently awake. She repeats the Fall from paradise by eating the poisonous apple. The human soul wakes to earth-consciousness after a time, but the pure spirit form which is cherished and guarded in the realm of the etheric becomes benumbed. It now requires higher powers to lead it to an awakening in the spirit, for that is beyond the gnomes. They may only keep watch over the immortal part of the human being when it sinks into the sleep of the senses. They guard the eternal spirit-being of man for its Awakener.

5

Secrets of
the seasons

Once a human soul breaks through to the realm of the elemental beings, it begins to unravel the mysteries of coming-into-being and passing-away. The seasons and their rhythms speak more and more clearly to it, revealing the character of the changes that take place from summer to winter. When men invaded these realms as conquerors, using the forces of nature for their own purposes, the experiences symbolized in the ancient seasonal festivals faded away. The extent to which summer and winter were distinct spiritual experiences is now scarcely comprehensible to us, so removed are we from nature. In the seasonal rhythm, people experienced the laws of growth in themselves and the cosmos. They felt an expansion of their being with the sprouting and flowering of the plant world; and in autumn as the seeds formed they withdrew into themselves.

This was an experience between the poles of sense-life and thinking-life. The extent to which one or the other took the lead prescribed the soul-life of a humanity closely interwoven with nature. The alternation was between the crystal-clear element of thinking, turned within, and the colourful, expansive life which opened out in the joy of the senses to the world. In the language of fairy-tales these two poles of the soul's existence were called Snow White and Rose Red, and they were felt as two particular beings influencing the inner life.

In fairy-tales, experiences which are played out on the border of two epochs are often preserved: old faculties are caught before they vanish and the new, youthful soul-forces come in. When the soul recalls the time when it was still united with the spiritual world it views present conditions as if widowed. Thus the soul becomes a "poor widow" reduced to living alone. But then she remembers the forces germinating within which must be cultivated. "In front of the hut there was a garden with two rosebushes growing in it, one bearing white roses and the other red roses. She had two children who resembled the two rosebushes, and one was called Snow White, the other Rose Red."

The way in which the two children are described is an illustration of how the fairy-tales reveal the deeper life forces. Snow White is gentle and quiet and likes best to help her mother with the housework. Rose Red prefers skipping about the fields looking for flowers or catching butterflies. Hand-in-hand the children go through the world, and the mother tells them: "What one of you has, she must share with the other." Thinking and observing always have to consider each other. The ordering and the receptive powers of the soul complement each other. This difference between thinking which turns inward and observation which opens to the world, is reflected in every detail. Thus the mother says in the evening: "Snow White, go and bolt the door," and on the other hand: "Quick, Rose Red, open the door. It must be a wayfarer in need of shelter."

The fairy-tale describes an event clearly recognizable as a spirit experience, taking place in deep winter. In the evenings the mother, sitting with the children in the house with the door bolted, reads aloud while the little girls spin. Close by lies a lamb, and a white dove sits on a perch. These are their house companions. This is a picture of the devotion of the human soul to the Christ. What follows is an imaginative experience of the world's hidden forces with which the soul can connect during deep-winter meditation. There is a knock at the door and when Rose Red opens it, a bear appears. The children are terrified, the lamb bleats, the dove flutters until the bear begins to speak and the children become used to its presence. Fear at first overwhelms the soul on meeting supersensory powers for it must learn to understand the language of the spiritual world. After this, every evening, the bear is the trusted guest of the household, until in spring he leaves. As he goes out he is caught by a hook in the door which tears his fur. Snow White thinks she sees gold shining through the tear.

In lectures on old experiences of the seasons,* Rudolf Steiner describes how, in summer, human beings were so wholly surrendered to the cosmic light and warmth that they scarcely felt their own bodies. They experienced a gentle withdrawal in the days of the summer solstice, and only towards winter, when contracting forces began again to take effect in the earth's atmosphere, did they feel the pull of gravity. It was as though they were once more drawn back into the body. With inner perception they saw dark fear-some figures rising from the earth's depths. Among northern people, the midwinter mysteries were spe-cially celebrated and it was the custom to bring out masked figures which inspired fear and asked riddles. Initiates, however, experienced something deeper. Most of all in the Holy Nights, when the earth is

* *The Cycle of the Year*. (1923). Anthroposophic Publishing, London 1956.

interpenetrated with forces of crystallization, it becomes a reflection of the starry worlds. The heavenly forces streaming down from the zodiac are received by the earth and radiated back. At this time of year certain people could observe the heavens working in the earthly realms. They were confronted with the figures of the zodiac and other fixed stars as though they were shining up out of the darkness of earth. In them they recognized the powerful formative forces which create the human body. It is out of the wide expanse of the cosmos — so they felt — that the forces flow which built the "heavenly wain" which carries the soul down to earth. But this heavenly vehicle is taken hold of by the dark material forces of the earthly realm. Clumsily, and with a "thick hide" we grope our way down into our physical body. The heavenly wain in which we are borne becomes a bear. We are "confined and shrivelled into man," as Goethe said.

The Great Wain (or Great Bear) circling the Pole Star, was specially venerated by the northern folk. It was as though within it the mystery of the whole circle of the zodiac was contained — the circle that swings in harmony round the axis of the Pole Star. In the Finnish epic, the *Kalevala,* the sun, moon and stars come to woo the proud king's daughter. But the virgin human soul rejects them all, she will have only the North Star: "Him, by seven stars surrounded, his companions eternal." Together with the seven gleaming stars of the Great Wain, the Pole Star was venerated by the northern peoples as the image of the most sacred life-forces. But when, at midwinter, the wain was reflected from the depths of earth, it appeared to the seeing eye as a great bear. Now we can understand why Snow White sees a golden gleam through the tear in the bear's fur. We understand, too, when they tease the bear by tugging his fur or walking on him, the bear's warning cry: "Snow White and Rose Red, you'll beat your suitor till he's dead." For the Pole Star, and with it the star-picture of the Great Wain or the Great Bear, figure in the Finnish epic as the wooers of the virgin human soul.

The bear leaves Snow White and Rose Red in the spring to protect his treasure from the bad dwarves who appear in summer and hide whatever they can steal in their caves under the earth. Here we see conflict between the bear and the lower egotistic intellect. The fairy-tale describes how, despite being warned, the children always come unwittingly to the dwarf's assistance in his thefts. The human soul stands between bear and dwarf and serves the dwarf without any idea of the consequences.

Previously we met the elemental beings from a different perspective where the dwarves appeared as helpers of mankind. They are almost entirely of a head nature and this has a double significance. They were wise before man fully awakened in his intellect and as guardians of ancient spirit light could light the path into the etheric world where man could not enter without their help. But as beings of a head nature the gnomes succumb to the cosmic forces that tend to harden, for they are egotistic and soulless in their bright intellectuality. The dwarf in fairy-tales is not just a symbolic figure, for we are always dealing with actual beings of various kinds. There are gnomes who long for warmth of soul, and therefore admire the human self because it bears within it the faculty of love: the "Three Little Men in the Woods" and the seven dwarves of Snow White for example. But there are also gnomes who attack the heart forces who must be identified and ejected if human development is not to suffer injury. Once the dwarf has been overcome, the king's son can cast away his bear's skin and lead Snow

White to his kingdom, for he has been turned into a bear by the dwarf.

The soul's journey from the realm of nature into "the town" is depicted in three stages in the fairy-tale. The impoverishment of nature is completed, stage by stage, by the wicked dwarf: through his victory of the cold clever intellect the world is facing godlessness. Thus as Snow White and Rose Red walk to town to buy needles and thread they encounter the dwarf for the third time. He is struggling with an eagle on a rocky heath and, naively, they go to his assistance. The human intellect is so ready to decide for the dwarf against the eagle!

Only on their way home does the event take place that sets them free: the bear overpowers the dwarf, who sits gloating over his treasure. Immediately the noble prince is released from the bear's skin: the heavenly man, born of starry forces, awakens from earthly darkness to his true nature. The newly won spirit-treasures of the earthly world shine out for him and he re-enters nature as his kingdom.

Musäus, in the fairy-tale the "Stolen Cloak", tells of the marvels of St John's Eve. He describes the daughters of man in whose veins still flowed "a drop of etheric blood". From a fairy grandmother the daughters have inherited the capacity to change into swans. They are swan-children, like Helen, the daughter of Leda. The daughters of Leda do not, like other human children, enter the world naked, for their bodies are covered with a kind of airy garment woven from densified etheric light-rays which expands as they grow. It has all the characteristics of the pure fire-ether, enabling its wearer to overcome earthly gravity and fly to the clouds and beyond.

There are three fountains where the swan-maidens

fly every year to rejuvenate themselves in the holy waters: in Africa, the sources of the Nile; in Asia, a lake at the foot of Mount Ararat; in Europe, the swan-pool in the western foothills of the Sudeten mountains. A Swabian knight named Friedbert, who has lost his way after a battle, meets an old hermit by the swan-pool and is initiated into these mysteries. Friedbert changes his knightly armour for the simple cloak of a hermit and waits year after year at the pool until, one St John's Eve, he surprises the maidens bathing in the pool and steals from one a swan-cloak and golden crown. Unable to fly home with her sisters, she is left with the hermit. He takes her for his bride, but the day before the wedding Friedbert's mother, having no idea of the maiden's origin or her mysterious power, gives her the cloak which her son has hidden. The maiden dons it, changes into a swan and flies out of the window. Only after many trials and journeys does Friedbert succeed in winning her again from the Orient, where she has been living as a princess.

When a swan is mentioned in fairy-tales or sagas it always refers to the heavenly part of the human being. He who can turn into a swan is able to awaken the innocent forces of his being, and rises into the pure etheric worlds out of which he descended before birth. (The image of the stork which carries the infant child to its parents is a similar imagination for the heavenly forces which guide us from pre-natal existence into earthly life.) He who regains his swan-wings experiences his origin in the light and feels all the more painfully how far man has strayed from his true nature. Only when the paradise nature is born again within, can man gain full knowledge of the facts of the Fall from paradise. These were the experiences that initiates underwent during the summer solstice mysteries when the soul soared into the cosmic ether and saw, in mighty images, the origin of the human race from the heights of the sun.

The possibilities of experiencing this upsoaring become more remote as mankind plunges deeper into materialism. Souls have become too earthbound: they have lost their swan-cloaks. Few still feel in their veins that "drop of etheric blood". In fact, as Musäus shows, a special quality in the blood is necessary for the unfolding of such soul-forces. The swan-maiden Friedbert sees on St John's Eve is the virgin ethereal part of his own soul. When he is empowered by the "cloak", he is able to celebrate the marriage with his "eternal-feminine". But the fairy-tale shows also how difficult it is to hold on to such an experience. The spirit powers won by Friedbert in the loneliness of his own soul are wrested from him. The knight has to follow quite new ways in order to win the swan-maiden again: ways which demand courage to face death.

The ancient mysteries of the summer solstice, which sprang from the northern pagan wisdom concerning nature, have lost their force. Mankind needs new ways to the spirit. Life must be reborn out of death. The Christian feast of St John is not regressive for we can now celebrate it with the powers of a renewed Christianity. It is a festival of awakening to remind us that we have lost our swan-cloaks with which at one time we could arise, free from guilt, to ethereal heights. It will arouse the longing to seek in new ways for all that has been lost.

The Christian mysteries guide the soul from midsummer, with its wealth of sense perceptions, into midwinter when the crystalline forces radiate down from the periphery, and the pure Snow White nature can be born in the soul. The fairy-tale of the "Juniper Tree" takes us into that same mood of inspiration which comes to the earth when the snow falls. With a magic of its own it describes the nine months of waiting. By following with sympathy the events of the seasons the mother experiences the ripening of her own fruit until in autumn she bears her child. This rhythm of the waiting-time is woven in with the arrangement of the festivals in the course of the year: that which descends from heavenly heights in the time of the Holy Nights can be nurtured as a seed in the soul-life and carried inwardly until at Michaelmas it is ripe to appear in the world. It can appear as will force and become active on the earth in Christlike deeds.

The brothers Grimm placed at the end of their collection the short fairy-tale the "Golden Key". It tells of a poor youth who goes out in the deep winter snow to fetch wood on his sledge. Almost frozen with the cold, he tries to light a fire and discovers a little golden key. Digging deeper, he finds an iron casket which the key fits. He puts the key in and begins to turn. "And now," — so the tale ends — "we must wait until he turns it all the way and opens the lid. Then we will know what marvels there were in the box." The situation described in the story corresponds to a turning-point in time. In this picture of the poor boy who stands in the cold and lights a fire in the snow, is there not portrayed the fate of Western Christendom, of Western mankind? The wealth of revelation in the old life of nature is over; the world is cold and the soul has become lonely. But the depths of winter hide a mystery. Where the heart lights a fire to enkindle the world again, there it also finds the key to new life-secrets. The Christmas festival provides holy warmth of the soul in the winter nights. It presents the golden key. "The key is there!" the fairy-tale is saying. And for he who digs deeply enough the treasure-chest is also there. But the new treasures are not yet open to view. The human soul knows the new direction for it has received the Christ mystery. But it does not yet know what sort of forces for the future are hidden within as it stands at the very beginning of the Christ revelation. And the soul must not forget, in the joy of having found the key, to uncover the treasure. The new wisdom, which is apocalyptic, will then begin to unfold itself and it has much, as yet undreamt of, to disclose.

6
The "Juniper Tree"

A fairy-tale which might have seemed to the brothers Grimm a model, a prototype, when searching through the endless files of their work, is the Low-German tale of the "Juniper Tree". They got it from Arnim who, in turn, obtained it from the painter Philipp Otto Runge who had heard it in his north German home together with the tale of the "Fisher and his Wife". Where the juniper trees grew on lonely heaths, standing like silent masked figures waiting for someone to probe their secrets, there were still people entrusted with old nature wisdom. Pictures of rare beauty were woven into their souls and these provided answers to the riddles of existence.

Voices of the invisible ones whispered from the dark silent juniper. The juniper was regarded as a rejuvenating tree. Its branches once crackled in the fires on the sacrificial altars of Germanic priests and its wonderful fragrance rose up to the gods. A mystery, guarded in the initiation centres of venerable Druids, was contained in the pictures of the fairy-tales.

On the heath "under the juniper tree" the neo-phytes ready to devote themselves to the ancient Druid wisdom were instructed. The priestly guides set them difficult and painful tasks in order to transform the lower personality and release the spiritual self from its coverings. For the soul this meant cutting into the quick of life as if with sharp steel, for if the self was to be freed from the chains of sense-perception earthly feelings had to be sacrificed and "blood must flow". But the wisdom imparted, which sank into the pupil's soul with crystalline clarity, could come to life inwardly only if it was shot through with warmth of feeling. The life-warmth had to be offered up to the pure world of thought. Eventually this activity of soul became a spiritual vision for the pupil. His soul, dedicated to striving after knowledge, was revealed to him in the form of a woman standing in the midst of a wintry landscape. She carried in her hand the fruit plucked from the tree of paradise, which man bore within him as the egotistical self. As she peeled the apple she cut her finger with the knife and blood flowed, gleaming in the snow. Thus it dawned upon the pupil that a higher, purer ego would be granted him as a gift of the spirit when the knowledge he had gained became glowing life. "Ah," sighs the woman in the fairy-tale, "if only I had a child as red as blood and as white as snow."

The image of the drops of blood shining in the snow served as a sign that the mystical evolution of the soul had begun. We meet this imagination in the Grail saga, as well as in the story of Snow White. Chrétien de Troyes describes how Perceval rides out one morning and comes near King Arthur's court. He crosses a snow-covered meadow where a flock of geese fly up. A falcon seizes one, wounding it in the neck. The bird escapes but three drops of blood fall as it flies away. When the knight sees the blood in the snow, he has a vision of his distant beloved, Blanchefleur.

The images of the Grail engendered a particular form of Christianity in the Middle Ages. From Ireland it was carried by Irish and Scottish missionaries into Europe. There it bore fruit in mystery centres and works of Christian charity, until the power of the

Roman Church overwhelmed it. This Christianity, nourished from the old Celtic wisdom, was based on direct supersensory experience and could witness the Christ deed without recourse to historical tradition. The significance of this Celtic mystery-cult was described repeatedly by Rudolf Steiner. There were places in Ireland where the Mystery of Golgotha was experienced directly through spiritual vision at the same time as it took place in the Holy Land. The Celtic initiates and their disciples knew of the penetration of the earth's being by the Christ without Bible or apostolic missions. For centuries this Hibernian Christendom flourished until it was eclipsed and supplanted by the Roman Church. In the legends of Saint Bridget (or Saint Bride) a further glimpse of such experiences can be found. Brought up by the Druids, the maid one day found herself carried in the spirit to distant lands, where she attended the birth of the Saviour.

Above all, however, the search for the Holy Grail, the vessel gleaming with the blood of Christ, continued far into the Middle Ages to light the path to the mystical experience of the Mystery of Golgotha. It is a mystery of the blood, and to imaginative contemplation it appears as the ripening of new forces rejuvenating life and transfiguring nature.

Wherever the folk-soul came into contact with this stream of Celtic Christianity — as happened from the seventh and eight centuries in the whole of Western and Central Europe — this Christ-light can be found in the imaginations that arise in legends and fairy-tales. Thus we touch on the inner sanctity of German folk-lore, for it was born out of a culture into which a hidden spirit-light shone. Although some motifs can be traced to the East or back centuries before Christ, the dismantling of fairy-tales into their mere motifs is like reducing a poem into its single sounds. We must look to inner imaginative logic if we are to penetrate the realms of experience from which the imaginations originate.

"A long time ago, at least two thousand years, there was a rich man who had a good and beautiful wife, and they loved each other dearly," the "Juniper Tree" begins. The life of those who follow the path of the soul becomes a legend which starts, in this case, with a man rich in treasures of ancient wisdom and a wife whose soul is filled with piety. The soul burns with longing for the life of the higher self — the birth of the spirit-child. But if the true self is to be born a sacrifice must be made. "If I die, bury me under the juniper tree," the woman tells her husband in the eighth month of pregnancy. After the child's birth, she dies happy and is buried under the sacred tree.

The human being belongs to two worlds: the earthly world in which destiny places him with his sense-nature — the "second wife" who also bears a child — and a higher world from which the new individual comes to birth under the sacred juniper tree. Along with the spirit inspired, a consciousness develops that falls into guilt and error through ignorance. The higher self finds it difficult to live with the sense world and must suffer persecution and scorn and finally, as we discover in the fairy-tale, even death.

The "Juniper Tree" tells of a little child — the holy child with no earthly name — and his half-sister, Marleenken. The sister, who shares the wicked mother's guilt and longs to atone for the child's beheading, bears a form of the name of the great penitent, Mary Magdalene. Thus the fairy-tale points to a deep connection between its images and the characters in the Gospels but its imaginations arise from direct contemplation of spiritual processes, rather than biblical reports.

The Golgotha of the innocent child is vividly portrayed. It is an inner way of the Passion and takes place whenever the child-forces of the soul are abandoned to an intellect chained to the senses. The stepmother is possessed by evil powers. When her daughter asks for an apple, the mother tells her she must wait till the boy comes home from school. When he returns, she entices him to the pantry and as he reaches into the apple chest the devil prompts her to slam the lid down and decapitate the boy. Terrified, she tries to shift the guilt to her daughter. The stepmother puts the head back on the body and places the boy by the door with an apple in his hand. Marleenken is sent to ask for the fruit. When he doesn't respond she slaps the boy's face — as her mother bids — and the head falls off. She weeps bitterly as the mother chops the boy up and makes him into a stew. The father is dejected when he returns and discovers his son is not home but cheers up as he eats the delicious stew, tossing the bones under the table. The girl carefully collects them, wraps them in a silk cloth and carries them, weeping, to the juniper tree. "Then the juniper tree moved; its branches parted and came together as though it were clapping its hands for joy. A mist went up from the tree, in the middle of the mist was a flame, and out of the flame rose a beautiful bird that sang gloriously and flew high into the air." The girl goes home merrily, as if her brother were still alive.

In order to understand the story's deeper connections with the Christian mysteries, we must focus on specific aspects. Christ set a child in the midst of the disciples to show them: "Unless you become like children, you will never enter the kingdom of heaven." The openness to higher realms which is natural in childhood is shut off when the earthly intellect awakens. In the Gospel of Matthew (18:3–6) we read: "Whoever causes one of these little ones to stumble, it would be better for him to have a millstone fastened round his neck." When the young boy returns home from school one day, he is ensnared to the chest. If the child develops only his everyday intellect, his immortal being meets death at Golgotha, the place of the skull.

Whatever spiritual power the magic of a happy childhood awakens in us must first make its way through the life of the sense-world. It must pluck the fruit of the Tree of Knowledge: reaching for the apple means delivering oneself up to the death forces of matter — the wicked stepmother. We encounter this fact but are not quite able to grasp how the once living spirit has incurred death, and our soul may feel guilty on that account, mourning the loss of the divine childlike part of its being.

The living forces of the spirit, when dimmed to a shadow in the intellect, take refuge in the deeper nature of the human being. The "flesh and blood" of the divine Son become, unconsciously, the spirit's nourishment. The dead remains of the spirit — our benumbed earthly intellect — awaits revival on a higher level. It must be brought into contact with the dead mother in the depths of feeling through a mystical awakening, for this divine part can celebrate its resurrection only when the death of the divine-spiritual within is experienced with the utmost intensity of which earth-bound consciousness is capable.

Under the sacred tree where "the good and beautiful wife" is buried, the dead thoughts, the bony remains of the child, can be revived and awakened. Then the intellect, ensouled with the force of religious devotion and once more connected to the primal powers from which it sprang, can be fully spiritualized.

Thus Good Friday and Easter become facts of a mystical soul development, as once they were earthly historical events. The power of thought, awakened to supersensory life, now appears in spirit-form to the human soul, announcing its own secret as an eternal Gospel:

> My mother killed me,
> My father ate me,
> My sister Marleenken
> Gathered up my bones,
> Tied them in a silken kerchief,
> And put them under the juniper tree.
> Keewitt, keewitt, what a fine bird am I!

The announcement to mankind by the miraculous bird takes place in three stages. As it flies to the goldsmith's workshop, the shoemaker's house and the clattering mill, we can see in each of its destinations a reflection of the development of Christendom.

The goldsmith making a golden chain in his shop is first to be summoned by the power of the bird's song. He hurries out into the bright sunlit street and begs the bird to sing again; but in exchange he must give the golden chain. Souls who preserved the golden chain of ancient wisdom were the first to meet the Christ-mystery with understanding. Their longing for the light was so strong that they could leave everyday matters to follow the call of the spirit.

But Christianity had to learn to stand firmly on the earth. The shoemaker hears the resurrection song and has to shield his eyes against the blinding light in which the bird hovers. He is more closely bound to the earth and so more capable of love. He calls his whole household out to participate in the liberating message. Not mysticism striving for personal revelation, but an energetic helpful Christendom, a community life, is pictured. The shoemaker gives the bird red dancing shoes.

Proclaiming the resurrection message is no light task in the turmoil of the machine age. Twenty boys sit in the clattering mill making a heavy millstone. Slowly the bird's song penetrates the deafening noise of the workshop and one by one they stop working and listen. As the final notes fade away, the last of them is ready to hear the message. But the bird asks for the heavy millstone in payment. The stone, which crushes and grinds the vital grain, should be borne aloft in the light of the resurrection, but this cannot be done by one man alone, however willing. Only when everyone is ready to devote their work in the material world to the spirit is it possible to hoist the stone. The bird puts his head through the hole and, wearing the stone like a collar, flies back to the tree and sings his song again. The redemption of the earth can begin only with the sacrificial deeds of mankind.

The fairy-tale ends with a powerful picture of the Last Judgment. As the bird sings from the roof of its parent's house, the father feels warm streams of sunlight and a deep inner joy. The mother experiences fear and Marleenken weeps for her lost brother. One after another they leave the house to listen to the spirit-message. The father joyfully accepts the golden chain and Marleenken skips and dances when she is given the red shoes. Lastly, full of fear, the wicked stepmother goes out and is crushed by the stone hurled down by the bird. This judgment illustrates the separate but interwoven forces working within human nature. The primal human being is again gifted by the spirit with the lost wisdom; the grieving soul learns how to overcome the weight of earth; but the sense-nature falls victim to the dead weight of matter, whose servant she has become. Finally the miracle-bird changes back into its child form, rejuvenated like the phoenix which has always been seen as an ancient foreshadowing of the mystery of Easter.

At the end of the story, the Saviour stands again before the spiritually awakened, as brother of the human soul. "He took his father and Marleenken by the hand, and they were all very happy, and they went into the house and sat down at the table and ate," the tale ends. Through these pictures of the judgment, one can feel the words of the Revelation of St. John resound: "Behold, I stand at the door and knock; if any one hears my voice and opens the door, I will come in to him and eat with him and he with me."

Although whispers of ancient wisdom from Celtic-Germanic mysteries are hidden in the fairy-tale, it can be seen as a Christian mystery of transformation. It all happened a long time ago "at least two thousand years", the story says. It might be transporting us to the beginning of our era, but it does not present allegorically the events in the Holy Land. Wherever there is a genuine quest for the spirit, these same events can be inwardly experienced. For then, as Richard Wagner could say of the Grail event, "time becomes space". The death and resurrection of Christ are felt each time the sacred story arises anew in the human soul.

7

Brothers and sisters

We have become acquainted with the double nature of
the human being in the images of folklore: in "Snow
White and Rose Red" it is represented by the two
sisters, in the "Juniper Tree" by brother and sister. An
inner conformity with natural law dictates the gender
of fairy-tale characters. A male represents the active
side of human nature. He will take the form of a king's
son if creative spiritual activity is illustrated, or in any
calling where an active direction of the will is required.
But if a naive spiritual striving is indicated he may be
depicted as a boy or youth. The passive receptive side
of human nature is shown as female: sensitive deep
understanding as a mother; lower knowledge bound
up with the senses as a stepmother; the pure
unawakened consciousness which can open up to
wisdom as a young girl, or, if already illumined by
wisdom, as a king's daughter with golden hair.

Little Brother took his little sister by the hand and
said: "Since our mother died, we haven't had a happy
hour. Our stepmother beats us every day, and when
we go to see her, she kicks us and drives us away ... let's
go out into the wide world together," begins the tale of
"Little Brother and Little Sister". Thus the human
being, no longer feeling at home in the world of the
senses, goes out into "homelessness". This escape of
the soul from all it has trusted into the borderland

between the sense-world and the spirit-world, is represented in fairy-tale images as a journey into a great forest. Here, where there are no clear paths leading to a sure goal, the soul encounters loneliness and the possibility of error.

Dante's *Divine Comedy* also begins with this borderland experience. The lost wanderer in the wood meets three beasts who bar his way: lynx, lion and wolf threaten his life. They are often taken allegorically to stand for sensuality, pride and avarice but one can do justice to such images only by referring to the sphere of experience from which they originate. Only what is illumined by knowledge appears in supersensory realms as a human form and the unconscious forces in human nature, the impulses and passions, take on animal forms. The more the soul is dependent upon a passion, the more threatening and bloodthirsty appears the corresponding beast. This is also true in the realm of dreams.

Little Sister cautions her brother when he wants to drink from enchanted springs bewitched by their wicked stepmother. "If you drink of me, you'll be turned into a tiger," murmurs the first spring; "if you drink of me, you'll be turned into a wolf," says the second. The tiger would tear the sister to pieces and the wolf devour her. Prudence may master desire and self-seeking, but not the general joy of the senses, the urge towards experience and adventure. The boy finally quenches his thirst at the third spring, which changes him into a fawn. Little Sister weeps, but she knows how to guide the fawn. She ties her golden garter round his neck and leads him with a soft rope made of rushes. They make their home in an empty hut and spend the days gathering nuts, roots and berries to eat. When desire-nature is led by the soul's wisdom, the human soul can live in healthy inter-

change between receptiveness to the world and consciousness of self. Every evening, satiated and wearied
with sense-impressions, it may return again to itself.

One day a great hunt attracts the fawn and Little
Sister reluctantly lets him participate. The fawn is
wounded, and the king follows him back to the hut and
asks the girl to come to the palace and be his wife. Little
Sister is overjoyed but insists that the fawn accompany
her.

The world of the senses is under the power of death-
forces; yet only where death-forces are active can
consciousness develop. These death-forces, which are
there to awaken knowledge, appear in the form of the
hunter. We would never find our way out of the forest
of superabundant nature if there was no death in the
world. It is not only at the end of our earthly existence
that death effects an awakening of the soul to the
spirit, for all our consciousness during life unfolds
through the dying processes in the organism.
Through supersensory observation of the human
being we know that these forces are fundamental,
especially for the opening out of the life of knowledge.

Little Sister marries the king and gives birth to a
baby boy, but the stepmother suffocates her and foists
her one-eyed daughter on the king. At midnight the
soul of the dead queen appears, feeds her child and
caresses the fawn. The king, watching this phe-
nomenon, recognizes the apparition as his true wife
and she is restored to life. The witch and her daughter
are judged, and when the witch is burned to death, the
fawn recovers his human form.

Fairy-tales often describe how the goal of the path of
suffering is not yet attained with a royal wedding.
When the soul receives the gift of spirit-powers, a
higher consciousness is born: a seed which must be
cultivated to bear fruit. But there is a danger that

human nature, not yet purified from all sense-inclinations, will allow the lower forces to come into untested connection with the higher consciousness. Once the soul is awakened to the spirit, it must develop the power of judgment in order to distinguish atavistic soul-capacities from the new spirit-consciousness.

Whenever one-eyed figures appear, they indicate the original clairvoyant consciousness which was bound up with a human sense organ. Anthroposophy suggests that the pineal gland is the stunted remnant of that original organ of light and warmth through which the surrounding world was observed in a dreamy way. It was the "eye" of man in ancient Atlantis. The "one-eyed" oppose progress and try to return to old twilight forms of experience. Odysseus strives for an awakened conscious understanding; he burns out the Cyclops's primitive eye. In this way he triumphs over the ancient atavistic soul-state.

The fairy-tale figures in "One-eye, Two-eyes, and Three-eyes", place before us the stages of man's evolution. Two-eyes, because she looks no different from other people, is despised by her sisters. Souls which have lost the ancient clairvoyance seem, at first, inferior to those who have retained it. They are considered less gifted by the proud souls who have brought traces of the old capacities with them. The tale shows how Three-eyes, who represents a mingling of the old clairvoyance with the new sense-perception and intellectual capacities — a kind of transitional stage — is especially dangerous to Two-eyes. In One-eye the old visionary state now acts very dimly — she can be "put to sleep". In Three-eyes it works with the earthly intellect and is therefore more egotistic. But in Two-eyes, who has completely overcome the old condition, the forces of the future act positively. Only she can pick the fruit from the golden tree of life and win the king's son. Only through repudiation of decadent spirit-powers can the soul attain that clarity of conscious awareness which can unite anew with the life-forces of the ancient condition. Those who cannot free themselves from chaotic old capacities become destitute, for they cannot connect with the present.

Thus, in "Little Brother and Little Sister", the one-eyed daughter who tries to take the place of the queen has to be recognized by the spirit and driven out. Until that happens the wise soul, which has been thrust aside into the realm of night and keeps watch over the sleep of the new spirit-seed (the child) cannot find release. And the will-nature, which still bears unsatisfied sense-longings within itself (the fawn) can be freed from the fetters of its desire only when the earthly, self-seeking consciousness is purged in fires of purification. The spell is broken when the wicked stepmother is burned to ashes.

Another fairy-tale that glorifies sisterly loyalty is "Fledgling". Again it depicts a boy and a girl who journey into the world because danger threatens them in their father's house. But the background is significant. A forester finds a little child in the wood, sitting high up in a tree, weeping. The mother had fallen asleep, and an eagle had taken the child into the tree. The forester takes the child home to bring up with his own little Lenchen. We are reminded of the story of Marleenken, but in this case the foundling is called Fledgling indicating he is not quite of the human kingdom.

The tale reveals a mystery experience. The man who knows his way in the wood, where others habitually go astray, is an initiate. In the figure of the "forester" lives the guardian of the hidden spiritual knowledge. He hears the child's cry for help, and knows how the heavenly part of human nature is removed to higher worlds during the early years of life. Normally, this process takes place unconsciously. But the seeker of the spirit must retrieve this supernatural part and learn to relate it with everyday consciousness, the "sister".

Sanna, the cook, plans to kill Fledgling but Lenchen learns of the plot and, after pledging their loyalty, the two children flee through the dawn into the forest. When the cook discovers the empty beds, she sends three servants in pursuit. The children see them coming and transform themselves; Fledgling is a rose-bush and Lenchen a rose. Old Sanna penetrates the secret and sends the servants out again, but the children change themselves into a church and a crown. When the searchers have again failed Sanna sets out to find them. Meantime Fledgling is a pond and Lenchen a duck. As the old cook bends over to drink up the pond, the duck pulls her into the water and she drowns. Joyfully, the children return home.

The development of the heavenly nature of child-hood is threatened by egotism which lives in the warmth of the blood. The fire of the passions burns up the super-earthly part which has the power to bestow holiness on the child's soul. Whoever unites the supersensory power of the spirit in sisterhood with the soul must also come to recognize the earthly powers which are inimical to the life of the spirit. He must learn how the soul which has surrendered itself to the spirit begins to develop a consciousness beyond that of the body. Impressions of a quite new kind appear on the soul's horizon between sleeping and waking. But in the morning, at the moment of awakening, they are extinguished by the consciousness of the senses. In order to grasp these imaginative experiences from the realm of the night, the soul must awaken before plunging into the bodily nature. Thus Fledgling and Lenchen have to leave home before daylight to forestall Sanna.

But what is the soul's experience when it is united with the spirit? It begins to realize that it is not confined to the bodily form, for at night a transformation takes place and it surrenders its inner life to nature. Rudolf Steiner describes how at night our souls plunge with their recollections into the hidden weaving life of nature. Just as in sleep the self surrenders to the elemental world everything it had expressed in gesture and countenance during the day so the soul releases into the realm of natural phenomena its memories of the day. These experiences pour continually into the hidden forces of plant growth and crystal formation and in this way man enriches and renews the life of nature.

The rose, for instance, takes into its ethereal life the very earliest experiences of our childhood. How little we recall of these early impressions: the love and care that surrounded us, our awe at things as their significance began to dawn on us. All this builds us up and forms us into the beings we become, but then it sinks down into the unconsciousness and appears only as attitude or mood. From the purest memories of childhood, the rose receives its soft beauty and exquisite scent. And this is the reason why we have special regard for the rose. As the flowers and trees take up these memory pictures, their ethereal life is animated by the noble or lower experiences which emanate from the human soul during sleep.

To imaginative cognition the whole of nature reveals flowing spirit-life. The world of phenomena begins to become transparent: soul-life radiates out of its manifold forms. Our childhood with its pure magic may vanish but nothing is lost which was once perceived and experienced in our inmost depths. As though enchanted, behind the rose-hedge sleeps the likeness of our childhood days. In this etheric realm lies Brier Rose, the Sleeping Beauty, awaiting her awakener. The recovery of the pure nature of our childhood which, to use the fairy-tale image, was put to sleep by the prick of the spindle on its fifteenth birthday, is thus a mystery of awakening. It is connected with the purification of the blood. When the forces of love experience their sanctification, the human blood is transfigured. Within it arise new streams of life related to the pure formative forces of the rose.

In this light the transformation of Fledgling becomes comprehensible. Fundamentally, the lower senses are incapable of destroying the supernatural of the pure sense-life of childhood. They can only prevent it temporarily from active life in the body: Sanna forces Fledgling to flee the house. But the children pass over into the life of nature and the holy soul-forces of childhood are transformed into the blossoming rose-bush. Behind the rose the innocent powers of the soul weave their formative forces, preserved unharmed from all impurity. The earthly senses, which are only servants of the lower consciousness, can never grasp these nature mysteries. But the soul which is loyal to the spirit gains its royal status in other worlds. From now on, though persecuted on earth and with no enduring home, it can dwell in sacred spirit realms. Thus its true radiance shines out for it becomes a crown resting in the church.

But the soul still has to learn to move freely in supersensory realms. This involves the capacity to abandon the support of the sense-world and consciously exist in the midst of flowing spirit-forces: the duck swims on the waves.

The spirit has this capacity in itself. The soul that can trust itself courageously to life is borne up by its streaming and weaving pictures. The soul has left behind the world of defined objects and fixed ideas and can no longer be confined by earthly illusions. The wizardry of earthly sense-nature is eclipsed as soon as experience of the weaving spirit and its formative forces begins. But the supersensory consciousness, which the sense-nature has taken fully into itself and released, can now take up its dwelling again, in freedom, in an earthly house. The soul dares to give the spirit space. That which could formerly only live and weave in the realms of night can now appear in the awakened day-consciousness.

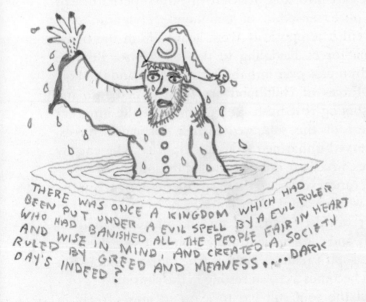

THERE WAS ONCE A KINGDOM WHICH HAD BEEN PUT UNDER A EVIL SPELL BY A EVIL RULER WHO HAD BANISHED ALL THE PEOPLE FAIR IN HEART AND WISE IN MIND, AND CREATED A SOCIETY RULED BY GREED AND MEANESS .... DARK DAY'S INDEED ?

8

Becoming human

To incarnate in a human body is an adventure. But life leads us into a dark magic forest where we can get hopelessly lost. It seems merciless how a young human being is thrust into an unknown, pathless, world. In the fairy-tale "Hansel and Gretel", we have exactly such a feeling. But just when the children feel sure they will die of hunger and weariness, a beautiful white bird appears and guides them to a little house in a clearing. And as they come closer, they realize that the house is made of bread, the roof is made of cake and the windows of sparkling sugar. Eagerly, they begin to nibble at it!

In Hansel and Gretel's action we see a parallel with the young human being working on its sleeping bodily vesture. The spirit weaves and works on the body, above all on the form of the head, to prepare it as a dwelling for itself. In the earliest years the child's skull is still pliable, and the essential self, a supersensory creative force, begins to model the head to its own design. It breaks open the roof, as it were, and with what joy does the soul press through to the experience of the senses. The story tells how Hansel breaks off a piece of the roof, while Gretel pushes out the window-panes.

"Nibble, nibble little mouse. Who's that nibbling at my house?" calls a soft voice from within. And the children answer: "The wind so wild, the heavenly child," and go right on eating, until the door opens and an old woman with a crutch hobbles out. After a grand meal they are ushered into two little beds; only to discover in the morning that they are really prisoners. Hansel is locked in a shed to be fattened up, for the witch plans to eat him. Gretel has to work and carry food for her brother, while she receives nothing but crayfish shells. The witch decides to eat Hansel, but Gretel pushes her into the oven where she burns to death. After filling their pockets with precious stones from the witch's house, Hansel and Gretel set out for home. A kindly white duck carries them across a lake, and once on the other side they see their father's house in the distance. The wicked stepmother, who had forced the children to wander in the forest, has died and their father is overjoyed to see them.

The human being is not solely the product of the stream of inheritance. What originates in father and mother serves the growing human being only to a limited extent, so the soul-spiritual being of man works on the body in the forming and ensouling of it. Thus we touch on the mystery of early child development, where a supersensory spirit-consciousness hovers, as it were, over the earthly body.

In religious writings the dove often appears as an image of the Holy Spirit. In fairy-tales, the pure spirit-forces, as yet untainted by the senses, are also symbolized by a dove or another white bird. As the "wind so wild, the heavenly child" plays around the earthly house to prepare a dwelling for itself, the dove hovers above. Supersensory life descends from the heavenly heights into the body. Here in an earthly body the spirit has to become aware of itself. It must receive nourishment out of the sense-experiences from the soul, so that it may grow and learn to hold the earth as its royal inheritance. But the little house is laid under a spell. Hansel and Gretel, whom we can regard as a duality of soul and spirit, wake up as prisoners in the witch's house.

Before long the immortal spirit forgets its goal. It falls asleep and is imprisoned in the growing child. Trapped within the body, it has to depend on the senses for nourishment, but the soul, allotted the task of maid-servant — Gretel forced by the witch to cook food to fatten up her brother — finds little satisfaction with this earthly world. The power which binds the spirit to the senses seeks to misuse, and ultimately destroy it. The old crippled witch — the intellect — is blind to the true nature and growth of the eternal in the human being. When the soul recognizes that destruction threatens the imprisoned spirit, purification of the hardened senses takes place: Gretel pushes the witch into the oven to die. The soul has rescued the immortal spirit from its bodily limitations and brother and sister can return united to their home.

Before they can achieve this however, a different state of consciousness is necessary. Those who travel towards the spirit experience that the earth is no longer firm under foot. To progress one must trust the stream of flowing life and travel on the wings of the spirit: the white duck takes Hansel and Gretel on its back. "And when they were safely across and had walked a little while, the forest began to look more and more familiar, and finally they saw their father's house in the distance." Once the spirit escapes the snare of the sense-world, it begins to recall the home from which it sprang.

Regarded from a spiritual standpoint was Hansel and Gretel's journey through incarnation a mistaken path? Not in its deeper sense, for the eternal being of man brings treasures of experience and knowledge back from life in the sense-world that can be acquired only in earth life. And this is characteristic of Western sentiment as reflected in its folklore: the progress of the human soul and spirit through earthly existence is fully affirmed. The human adventure is not a fundamental error as it can be regarded in Eastern wisdom. Incarnation is not merely suffering or guilt. Where the Christ light, consciously or unconsciously, gives sense and direction to earthly existence, our incarnation "adventure" takes a fortunate turn. Pearls and precious stones are borne to his father's house by the earthly pilgrim who travels the road to the spirit. Sense-existence begins to shower gifts on him the more consciously he masters it.

We need not conclude from what we have discovered that the same processes of thought had already been at work in the souls of those who first told tales such as "Hansel and Gretel". It is by no means a mere matter of clothing spiritual knowledge in symbolic forms. The true fairy-tale — if not in every detail of its repetition — is in origin directly traceable to imaginative experiences. But these experiences do not necessarily become fully conscious knowledge. In those intermediate states, representing a transition between waking and sleeping, the soul forces and their activity can be seen objectively, as though from outside.

Every night the supersensory part of man's being continues to try to ennoble and spiritualize the body. This work begins in our earliest childhood years when the higher ego forms the skull and sense organs so it can dwell in the body with its soul and spirit forces. Thus we come to describe the little house of cake more intimately: it is in fact not our physical body that the tale describes but a second body of formative forces — the etheric organism. On this our soul-spiritual being, when not living "at home" in sense-existence, begins to work in a conscious way. "Hansel and Gretel" is therefore a picture of the activity of a soul on the path to initiation; a soul occupied with the transformation of its hidden supersensory bodily nature into a vehicle of higher consciousness. This process is a continuation of the ego's work on the body in childhood. Whenever we fall asleep we return unconsciously to our life's own beginning and those who are spiritually awakened do so quite consciously. Thus the mysteries of childhood and initiation experiences are woven into the imaginations of fairy-tales.

The fairy-tales also reveal the sun mystery which preceded our descent into earthly existence. But in order to comprehend the human being's origin in divine light another realm of experience must be reached. Forms bearing the glint of a world far from earth must be carried over into the light of day-consciousness. Impressions of this comprehensive spirit-world are difficult to retain for the pictures die when they rise from the hidden depths and have to be captured by earthly thinking. At this stage of spiritual experience, a man can see himself as a fisherman on the sea-shore watching the dream realm vanish into the distance. As the great sea of night ebbs away from him, he feels bereft and poverty stricken.

It was as "fishers" that the men of old saw themselves when they tried to bring the bright dream pictures back from the depths of the night-world. The morning seemed to them like a long, slow return from the distant spaces of wave-tossed perceptions and weaving pictures, not as a sudden awakening into the body of the senses. Every time it was necessary to make a "landing". In the fact that the first disciples of Christ were called fishermen lies an indication that they were capable of bringing impressions from the spirit-world into day-consciousness. They achieved the "miraculous draft of fishes".

The old image of the fish stands for the innocent nature of humanity untouched by the earth and the fall into sin. A fish produces no warmth of its own and so feels itself as a part of its surroundings; it is one with the whole flowing sea. By contrast, warm-blooded beings are cut off and become egotistic. The Christ can restore to us the innocent consciousness which embraces the whole breadth of life. This is why in early Christian times he was often represented by a fish symbol.

In primeval times the being of man shone golden like the sun. Anthroposophy speaks of those times as the Hyperborean Age, when everything earthly was still impregnated with sunlike life. It is the Golden Age told of in the sagas. But only a reflection of this can be brought into our everyday life, for on earth the soul cannot live permanently with these forces. If the embodiment of our supersensory being is to be completed, that original sunlike consciousness must be dismembered. Only one part can be absorbed into earthly incarnation; its heavenly twin brother is left behind.

The story of the "Golden Children" indicates this. A poor fisherman catches a golden fish and is promised a magnificent castle if he lets it go. However, the fisherman must not tell how the castle with its inexhaustible cupboard of food has come into being. But since he cannot remain silent, the castle vanishes. Eventually the fish is caught and divided into six pieces: two of these are to be eaten by the fisherman's wife, two given to his horse, and two buried in the garden. Two golden children and two golden foals are born and in the garden two golden lilies grow. The twins grow up, and set out on the golden horses to discover the world. As long as they remain safe the lilies bloom but if harm befalls either brother the lilies wilt.

They come to an inn where the other guests insult them because they are "golden". One brother is overcome with shame and rides back to his father's house but the other has the courage to continue. To avoid falling into the hands of robbers in a great forest, he covers himself with bearskins. He rides through safely and arrives at a village where he meets, and marries, a beautiful girl. That night he dreams of a magnificent stag and in the morning sets out to hunt it in the forest. All day it eludes capture. At dusk, the twin comes to a witch's dwelling and is put under a spell. As he falls, petrified, to the ground his lily wilts in the fisherman's garden. Immediately the other brother sets out to find him, and forces the witch to disenchant his twin. They ride homeward, one to his waiting bride, the other to his parent's house where the two golden lilies stand tall and proud again.

Let us consider the starting point of such a fairy-tale. The poor fisherman grows immeasurably rich when he catches the fish. Suddenly, a castle with the miraculous cupboard of food stands in place of his hut. The contact with the "fish" awakens a deeper consciousness which, as the Greeks knew, lies under the diaphragm. Hidden in the solar plexus is the centre of that other nerve-system which penetrates our whole body and guides the nourishing processes in the organism. This sympathetic nervous system is imbued with a wisdom inaccessible to our ordinary consciousness. In this pure activity, untainted by personal control, sun-forces mingle and work in the unconscious building of the human body. Conscious access can be found to this activity in those special moments when the everyday consciousness is dampened. In such moments the soul can perceive the heavenly life-forces regulated from the solar plexus. The miraculous cupboard is opened: the mystery of the "table, spread thyself", known also in other fairy-tales, is played out before the awakened soul.

The motif of the enriched fisherman reminds one of the legends of the Grail. In the account by Chrétien de Troyes, Perceval is invited to be the rich Fisher-King's guest. In the shining castle of the Grail he is served a wonderful evening meal. The Grail does not endure any unnecessary mention of itself. Lohengrin, the envoy of the Grail, has to withdraw when asked where it has come from. Likewise, the castle with its lavish cupboard vanishes when the fisherman tells how it arose. Although it is not here a question of a Grail experience, both legends have a common factor. The shy forces from the depths have to withdraw before the grasp of earthly understanding. The intellectual impulse to ask questions darkens the light of that delicate comprehensive consciousness which has its seat in the sympathetic nervous system.

In the "Fisherman and his Wife", the miracle accomplished by the fish vanishes as soon as the soul overrides human limits and yearns to be "like God". It is Lucifer who insinuates a spirit of arrogance into human beings as soon as the old divine consciousness begins to fade away. Man tries to seize divinity, rather than open the way for the divine to take up its dwelling within by working on a progressive transformation of himself. Lucifer ruins the soul as the fisherman and his wife show when they end up living in their old pigsty.

The "Golden Children" tells the story in another way. It shows how the pure cosmic consciousness seeks to come as a gift to mankind. The golden fish decides to sacrifice himself: he is prepared to go through the process of becoming human. What the fisherman experiences as the birth and destiny of the two golden children reflects the history of mankind: our origin in the sun-worlds and descent into earth's darkness. A great sacrifice heralded the age when we begin to be individuals: a heavenly consciousness sent out from itself, in the act of dying, the twin forms of our humanity.

Old Hebraic wisdom spoke of Adam Kadmon, the cosmic primal human being. Paul's teaching differentiates between "the first and the second Adam": the first has entered the earthly world and become mortal; from him springs the earthly race of mortal man. The second Adam remained in heaven and only with Christ's coming descended to penetrate us with his immortal being. In him, the lost original image of humanity, preserved in its purity, seeks to bestow itself upon us again. That is the true meaning of our rebirth through the deed of Jesus Christ.

Once the urge towards earthly destiny awoke in the human beings living in the pure ethereal realms of paradise. They mounted the horse: they sought incarnation. But for that a separation had to take place. Only part of the light-filled human being can plunge down into the sheath of mortality to travel incognito — wrapped in "bearskin" — through the sense-world. The other, the more delicate part, draws back when the sun-gold is scorned. So he refuses incarnation and returns home where the lilies bloom. He decides to remain a child of heaven while his brother wanders the earth. The latter finds a bride: he burns for the earthly world and its beauty and is seized with an eagerness that will not let him rest. But when he has followed the chase all day in the forest of error he is turned to stone. His origin is forgotten and his guiltless heavenly counterpart is lost to him: the lily fades.

That is a consequence of incarnation. The sun-forces sent down to us unfold themselves as our selfhood. But, imprisoned in the earth, they forfeit their powers of light. The human being who has attained personality but is frozen within his own intellect no longer recognizes his real vocation and needs the help of the immortal counterpart. He descends to seek out the brother bewitched in the realm of transience, and thus becomes his awakener.

In the Greek legend, Castor and Pollux wandered over the earth. They were the sons of Leda, and Helen in whom the soul of Greece was adored was their sister. To the Greeks, the brothers represented the mystery of heroic manhood. Inseparable though the brothers were, their destinies were different, for Castor was mortal and Pollux immortal. When Castor received his fatal wound and descended to the underworld Pollux asked Zeus to make Castor immortal also. But that was contrary to cosmic law. It could only happen if Pollux would sacrifice himself and descend into the realms of death with Castor. Pollux made the great sacrifice and followed his brother to the world of the dead so that Castor might follow him into the realms of the immortals. Since then they live in the depths and the heights in turn — in continual coming and going.

The Greeks also looked up to the brothers in the winter sky. The constellation of Gemini, the Twins — the guiding light of all who wander in darkness, the trusted pilot for ships on the lonely waters — rise on winter evenings on the eastern horizon. Following it comes the bright star Sirius, venerated by all ancient peoples as the holiest star. Castor and Pollux appear like two heralds of the Christmas star. That we have here an ancient holy mystery motif is clear from the fact that the two brothers wander through the legends and fairy-tale literature of every country.

The most impressive tale of brothers is the longest story in the Grimms' collection. Called simply the "Two Brothers", it contains a wealth of motifs but here we shall deal with only one theme.

Every morning the brothers find a piece of gold under their pillow. They "sleep upon" the gold, as it were, bringing dream-wisdom into the day. The custom of sleeping on a difficult problem or decision arises out of a similar experience. Anyone who knows how to carry a thought through sleep, will find it again, enriched, in the morning. It returns from the realm of inspiration.

In the "Two Brothers", the two children of the poor broom-maker share this gift because they ate the heart and liver of a golden bird. Their father, instructed by his avaricious brother the goldsmith, shoots the bird from a tree with a stone. The goldsmith knows the bird's secret and wishes to gain the miraculous powers but these fall not to him but to the innocent children of the poor man. The gift of illumination dies if anyone tries to seize it for personal aims: the sun-inheritance of mankind does not allow itself to be drawn down by the earth's gravity. In the past, in moments of grace, inspired thoughts descended upon the soul: the golden bird let fall a golden feather, or left a golden egg in the nest. But self-seeking eagerness for the gold of wisdom drives it back into the spiritual realm of inspiration. It sinks into the depths of the soul, guarded in its innocence from earthly understanding. In the unconscious it becomes an active force which sends out its gifts of grace only from the realm of night, for in sleep the human soul is far wiser than in waking consciousness.

On the path through life the twin brothers have to separate: one goes east, the other west. In this we see a picture of mankind with Eastern man wandering

93

always towards paradise while Western man conquers the earthly globe and masters the world of matter. One soul cannot forget its origin in the light while the other has the courage to "venture out in the world" and is strengthened in personality: this is the twofold form of human striving. Towards the end, the fairy-tale strongly resembles the "Golden Children". The Western wanderer, despite heroic deeds and royal recognition, will ultimately become petrified in the bewitched forest. Release can come only with the help of the brother who went east. In the great migrations of mankind they were separated but they must come together again.

Raphael's picture *The Vision of Ezekiel,* shows the Christ breaking through the clouds as though surrounded by sun-powers. The Son of Man sinks in all the glory of his light down to earth, which lies under the darkness of storm-clouds. He is borne down on the shoulders of two youths: he needs both to enable him to appear on earth. An apocryphal saying has also come down to us: Christ, asked when his kingdom would come, answered: "When the two become one."

9

The cosmic mystery
of the twelve

Among the Grimms' legends for children is the
"Twelve Apostles", which tells of a poor widow who
can no longer support her twelve children. Forced to
send them out into the world to earn a living, she prays
to God to let her sons be on earth with the promised
saviour. The eldest son, Peter, lost in a dark forest,
finds a little boy "gleaming bright and as beautiful and
as friendly as an angel" beside him. After being led
into a crystal cave where twelve cradles lie side by side,
he becomes "like a little child," and the angel sings and
rocks him to sleep. One by one, the other brothers are
led to the cave by their guardian angels. They sleep
three hundred years until the night when the saviour is
born. "Then they woke and were with him on earth,
and were called the Twelve Apostles."

It was the son of a widow whom Elijah wakened
from death in the Old Testament story. This widow
also had no food for her son before the "man of God"
came to her. At the time, all who bore the pain of
earth's dark destiny felt themselves to be sons of an
impoverished widow. They perceived the withdrawal
of their ancient sacred inheritance of the spirit: the
bread of life for the soul was exhausted. The mystery
centres, which had guarded it, could no longer provide nourishment for mankind. All they could offer

95

was the counsel: "Study the earth, and wrest from it nourishment for yourselves!" In this search, humanity moved deeper into the earthly realms, unable to find an exit from the labyrinth, or food for their souls. Mankind had to plunge completely into experience of the body, and this meant the darkening of the higher being: it fell asleep in the crystal cave. The life of the spirit is paralysed in the crystalline forces of earth-bound thinking. Such is the entombment of human beings until the grave becomes a cradle.

By forfeiting its ancient wisdom and wresting the bread of life from the earth, the human soul is rejuvenated. Only when the soul is driven back into its inner life will it truly come to itself. This self is merely a sleeping seed until Christ comes to awaken it. Those human beings who followed the path into the earth's darkness cultivated in their souls a power which now, in a later life, needs only an awakening to come to fruition. When they meet the Christ they have the wondering gaze, the receptive hearts and a will for a new beginning, and so become his disciples. For they have regained the virtue of "becoming as little children".

The twelve apostles to whom the Christ first revealed himself must have been such souls. The fairy-tale implies that previously they had followed a particular path of soul-life in order to develop the necessary child-forces. This gives us a glimpse into the preparation for the appearance of Christ on earth and for Christianity: "Blessed are those who hunger, for they shall be filled."

These twelve figures appear in all sacred traditions of religion and folk legends as guardians of the original revelation and preparers for the way of the light. They appear in many guises from the twelve great Indian Bodhisattvas, said to descend in turn to the earth in order to raise humanity to their own heights, to the twelve knights gathered by King Arthur at his round table, who were sent out to perform valiant deeds. It was always twelve who had to unite in a common work for in the twelve, it was thought, the whole cosmic world was represented. This was held to be a valid cosmic law. Studying the Gospels in this light we see the twelve apostles as a reflection of the cosmic order — not simply as individuals, but as bearers of the cosmic powers which stream down from the twelve constellations of the zodiac.

Human existence — as a whole and individually — is born out of the twelvefold ordering of the starry heavens. From the Ram come different powers from those sent out by the Bull or the Fish. From them all, the twelve types of human beings receive their special imprints. The fairy-tale knows them as the eternal familiar brothers of every soul. There we find recounted their destiny, the enchantment they must endure and the hope of salvation through atonement by the soul.

The "Twelve Brothers" tells of a king who has twelve sons. He decides that if his thirteenth child is a girl, the boys must die so that she alone inherits the kingdom. Twelve little coffins are prepared but the grieving queen warns her sons and they flee into the forest. She promises to hoist a white flag if she bears a boy, or a red one to indicate a girl. They take turns watching the tower from the tallest oak and on the twelfth day, while the youngest brother keeps watch, a red flag is unfurled.

After vowing to avenge themselves on every girl who crosses their path, the twelve brothers flee deep into the forest where they find an enchanted hut. "We will live here, and you, Benjamin, because you're the youngest and weakest, will stay at home and keep house. The rest of us will go out and get food." Meanwhile the princess grows up "good of heart and fair of face" with a gold star on her forehead. She knows nothing of the twelve brothers who are homeless on her account until one day she finds twelve shirts among the linen. Full of guilt, she sets out into the forest to find her long-lost brothers.

In order to enter more deeply into a fairy-tale, it is helpful to start from the situation which indicates an awakening of the soul. A king's daughter who bears a golden star on her forehead is clearly destined for a spiritual awakening. Within her lives a knowledge which is not of the earth alone, for starlight irradiates her. When she discovers the hidden shirts her mother tells her the secret of her birth: there exists an ancient memory which can well up from the depths of the heart where it has been guarded through the ages. "My present consciousness," the awakened soul can say to itself, "has been dearly bought; for me to be queen, twelve other beings must be deprived of home and royal state. They existed before I did yet we are of the same origin, are brothers and sister." And the desire to find these royal powers can grow in the soul once it becomes aware of the guilt bound up with its cosmic existence. Here the fairy-tale touches on the mystery of the Fall from paradise.

There was a time when the human being had not yet gained a consciousness of self: when he was unable to speak of himself as "I". This consciousness lay dormant, but not yet severed from the etheric weaving of the cosmos as in the present condition of the world. Out of the twelve segments of the starry cosmos the formative forces worked together to build up the human form. And they worked again within the human form on the individual sense-organs. As through twelve doors, the life of the world in all its various manifestations flowed into the human being. There are twelve senses, the five familiar ones and seven duller, more elusive senses secreted deeply within the body — the senses of balance and warmth, for example.* The instinctive wisdom of older times conveys this knowledge in its own way: the senses are the "twelve brothers". Through the senses the world seeks to break into the soul's inner life. But there are difficulties. The flowing light seeks its entry and forms the human eye but the eye becomes a glassy coffin in which the divine light must first die in order to be given back to us as a shadow-picture. The resounding Word builds the human ear but the ear becomes a rocky cavern in which only the dead shell of the divine Word finds entrance.

A deep sadness can fall on the soul when it realizes the contrast between the potential of the senses and what they have become. They could be messengers; apostles of the glory of the Lord, collecting nourishment from all the realms of the earth for the coming into being of the human self, in order to bear the divine life through the twelve sense-doors into the depths of the soul. They are the legendary "apostles" who, as the turning point of time approached, were sent out into the world to seek nourishment. They were led to the crystal cave where they waited for the saviour of the world to awaken them. The legend thus gains a new background which harmonizes with the "Twelve Brothers".

* Rudolf Steiner lists the twelve senses as: sense of touch, life, movement, balance, smell, taste, sight, warmth, hearing, speech (perception of sounds as words), thinking (perception of the content of thought), "I"-sense (becoming aware of another's self, but not merely through empathy). While the lower senses, in their present form, merge into half-conscious body life the higher ones help us to grow beyond the narrow life of self. They are specifically human senses — especially the last which goes hand in hand with the coming into being of the human self.

In that tale, the royal cosmic powers which form the human body have to withdraw into the depths. The bewitched house in the forest (already encountered in "Hansel and Gretel") offers them hospitality. They cannot live in the warmth of the blood for that makes them egotistic. The "blood-red" flag which is hoisted after their sister's birth announces that there is no longer any room for the twelve in the earthly house. The cosmic formative forces must take refuge in a second, invisible organization which we bear within us. During daily life they remain unconscious, though continually active; building the human corporeality in mysterious ways and revitalizing it with etheric forces.

What we have retained in our bodies as senses are coffins in which true life no longer dwells. The soul is able to nourish a firmly established self only when the abundant life of the cosmos is dampened down. But this necessity implies a lasting impoverishment and limitation of the self for the awakened soul needs a dialogue with the cosmos and must try to regain its connection with the cosmic powers. Thus it ventures out to find the hidden life of the twelve brothers and finds them in the realms of etheric weaving. When the conscious eye of the senses fades during sleep, higher faculties of perception begin to rule and the world of the "brothers" rises before the imagination. In the fairy-tale, the princess finds the bewitched house in the evening. Benjamin questions her and realizes this beautiful girl is his sister. He talks persuasively to his brothers on their return and wins their favour for the princess. With what joy she is received! They live together harmoniously in the bewitched house for orderliness and purity reign when the king's daughter holds sway. But one day, in ignorance, the princess picks twelve lilies growing in the little garden in front of the house. The air is filled with rustling as twelve ravens fly off over the forest. She has bewitched her brothers who were the lilies.

In fairy-tales and religious symbolism, lilies indicate powers which are unwilling to merge with the earth; powers shy to incarnate. In contrast to the rose, which is strongly rooted in the earth and raises earthly matter to pure rose-essence, the lily forms a corm which is only loosely anchored to the ground. It is an image of virginity. Gabriel, the angel of the annunciation, is often portrayed with a lily because he comes from the realms of the unborn. Goethe's fairy-tale of the "Green Snake and the Beautiful Lily", also leads us into the world opposite that of the senses — the world of archetypal forms. The Lethe, the stream of forgetfulness, separates these two realms. In order to find his true archetypal self the king's son must cross over the stream. When we left that forgotten world to enter the snakes's realm our archetypal self remained behind in that land where the lily blooms.

In the fairy-tale of the "Golden Children", the lily dies when the brother it represents is turned to stone. In the midst of sense-existence he has lost the connection with his higher self. When the twelve lilies are plucked the hidden weaving of the higher senses is extinguished. The imaginative world becomes dark to the gaze of the soul once it depends upon earthly intelligence bound up with the sense-world. The old instinctive clairvoyance, active in humanity as long as certain innocent soul-forces remained over from the past, must die out altogether when the awakening intelligence of the soul-life begins to rule. In place of the lilies, ravens appear; instead of the quiet blossom, the whirr of ghostly wings. The cosmic senses must now lead a shadow-existence. The supersensory being of man is darkened within.

Lonely and guilt-ridden, the king's daughter remains in the forest of error. But the ancient wisdom knows the way of redemption. There have always existed bearers of higher knowledge who could show the way to the spirit. In the fairy-tale an old woman comes to the poor maiden and says: "My child, what have you done? Why didn't you leave those twelve flowers alone? They were your brothers, and now they've been turned into ravens forever." When the princess asks if there is a way to save her brothers, the wise woman answers: "You would have to keep silent for seven years."

Medieval Christianity knew the seven stages of the way of the Passion (from the Washing of Feet to the mystic Death and Resurrection) as the path of the soul to the awakening of the spirit. The human soul, ready for atonement, becomes the penitent disciple. In the sense of the Johannine teaching, the soul can experience again the Passion of Christ in the depths of its own being. Silence, the conscious withholding of the powers of speech, strengthens inner experience to an extraordinary degree. There is, however, a silence on a higher level: it is inner dumbness in the face of life's injuries, a readiness to meet the tests and trials of destiny as compensation for ancient guilt. The seven years, however, are not to be reckoned according to the calendar. They are years of the soul, and no day must be omitted if the silence is to have its redeeming effect.

The maiden, believing in her heart that she can do this, sits in a high tree and spins, neither speaking nor laughing. A king, while hunting, discovers her and sees the gold star on her forehead. He woos the dumb girl and leads her home as his bride. But because she keeps silence the wicked stepmother succeeds in persuading the king to condemn her to death. Just as the flames of the pyre kindle her clothing the seven years expire. A rustling is heard in the air; the twelve ravens swoop down, become the brothers again, and free their sister.

The fairy-tale describes how the soul meets with the higher self: the mystical wedding. In the language of Christian initiation, the human soul unites with the Christ. But at the same time as the soul is raised to the higher self it is sent to the stake, for its destiny is not to cause merely the destruction of the lower self, but its redemption. In accepting the flames — in taking them upon herself in silence — the young queen is also rescued from them. When she becomes free from the dross of self-seeking the twelve senses are released from the enchantment in the darkness of death. They rise from a shadow-existence into cosmic life. Through awakening the human being rediscovers the powers of his origin and grows out of his narrow self. Through the power of sacrifice he can expand to the cosmos.

The fairy-tale also portrays the cosmic development of the maturing human being. Before the child-being awakens to itself — before the "star" in it lights up — the child draws its life from the beneficent forces of the cosmos. The formative powers of the world which have built the body according to the laws of the stars withdraw, leaving behind the twelve "coffins" prepared for them — the earthly senses — as an image of their being. They carry on a hidden weaving existence which constitutes the magic of the child soul — its unconscious wealth and its dawning understanding of the world. At puberty, this magic is lost when, in unknowing guilt, the child sinks more deeply into the bodily nature. The lilies are plucked, the intellect is

darkened, the ravens rustle overhead. The redemption of the intellect can take place only through a
rediscovery of the forces of childhood. Creative cosmic
thoughts wait to celebrate their resurrection in the
ego.

Spiritual forces which have formed our senses out of
the cosmos and then have to withdraw when the
individuality awakens to a consciousness of itself
appear in the fairy-tales as brothers or princes. But if
the senses are regarded as powers of consciousness
waiting to be awakened they appear as twelve maidens.
This deeper view is taken, for example, in the fairy-
tale of the "Twelve Huntsmen". Twelve maidens
disguised as huntsmen come to the court of the king's
son who has forgotten his true bride. Only the wise lion
sees through the masquerade. He is the royal counsellor, the wisdom of the heart, which can see further
than the ordinary consciousness.

Innocent soul-forces, undimmed by the earthly
sense-nature and struggling to make themselves
known to the striving human being, at first appear in a
false form, as delusions before the human spirit. In
fairy-tales the forces of knowledge, in which there is
still present something of death, always take on the
appearance of hunters. The instincts of the soul-life
have to be condemned to death by the awakening
knowledge. In those who experience an awakening of
the heart, however, the intellectual forces of knowledge are transformed into intuitive ones. With these
transformed life-filled forces of wisdom the human
being can find his higher self if courageous enough to
reject the lower forms of knowledge. Loyalty to the
true bride — forgotten, but once more acknowledged
by the prince — is in fact loyalty to one's higher self

which was in danger of being lost in the world of ideas.

In the fairy-tale of the "Shoes that were Danced Through", a soldier seeks the answer to how the king's twelve daughters wear out their shoes each night. He discovers that they escape their locked room down a secret staircase and meet twelve bewitched princes. They cross a river, and dance all night in a glittering palace.

Here the fairy-tale points to a soul-mystery: there are cosmic forces, active in the night realm, which make the life of feeling too volatile. They separate the forces of the soul too much from the earthly bodily nature and waft them away to starry spheres. Those who lose themselves too far in the starry forces of the astral world at night run the danger of becoming less and less capable at their earthly tasks. With this inner wealth they return with a lack of interest in earth life and cannot find any joy in the experiences of the senses or display any energy for life's demands. Those who wear their shoes thin dancing all night cannot walk the earth securely and firmly during the day.

This condition of soul-life is quite common. It can also afflict people who seem wholly given up to fulfilling the duties of daily life. They may not be truly present with all their soul- forces or be able to put their whole heart into whatever they are doing. A civilization that has lost touch with its soul experiences increasing difficulty in bringing soul-forces into daily life.

The soldier in fairy-tale imagery is the human being who has to wrestle with evil forces and opposition in the development of his inner life. He penetrates with understanding into these inner spheres and wrests his soul-forces from the enchanted weaving of the astral worlds. The fairy-tale depicts the testing of the will. Man must find forces active enough to lead the complete human being back, strengthened into the body. As witness that he is able to stay awake in those starry realms, the soldier brings to the king a silver, a gold, and a diamond branch. He has learned to bring the holy forces of the cosmos back into earth-life.

10

Animals as
man's helpers

To unprejudiced observation it is evident that the whole of nature is permeated with creative intelligence. This weaving wisdom reveals itself differently in the plant and animal kingdoms. We can wonder at the wasp, who invented paper long before man began to manufacture it, or stand before an anthill and observe the intelligence which unites innumerable co-workers in the common will to build. Here a communal wisdom holds sway over the behaviour of each ant.

We have to acknowledge that there is ordered reason, as it were, poured over the whole group of creatures. We can imagine a realm of wise "group"-souls who stand behind each specimen of the animal species, continually sending them forth into the world. If we cultivate a reverential attitude towards these group-souls, it becomes possible for their wisdom to flow unnoticed into the soul. But in people whose tyrannical nature excludes this reverence, destructive rage can easily manifest. Not only in the technological exploitation of nature does this impulse reveal itself; we see it also in the child's desire to tear the heads off flowers or to break open anthills.

The "Queen Bee" tells the story of two sons of a king who set out in search of adventure. They fall into a wild, dissolute way of life and eventually the third brother, Blockhead, sets out to find them. They mock him for his simplicity but finally allow Blockhead to accompany them. They come to an antheap and the elder brothers want to root it up for entertainment but Blockhead prevents them. Next they plan to kill and roast ducks swimming on a lake: the third brother again intervenes. And when they discover a beehive and plan to take away the honey, Blockhead forbids them. Thus the brothers have wandered through three realms: earth, water and air. But only Blockhead has understood how to place himself in a moral relationship to these three worlds. He alone reveals the true wisdom of the heart. Likewise Perceval has to awaken in himself sympathy for the life of the animal world if he is to enter the realm of the "Grail". The compassion that makes him "world clairvoyant" must become allied with the purity of the fool.

The three brothers come to a bewitched castle where everything has turned to stone. They call out three times and a little grey man opens the door. Silently he leads them to a richly spread table, and when they have eaten he shows each to a separate bedroom. Next morning the little grey man shows them a stone tablet with an inscription of the tasks that have to be performed to break the spell. Anyone who fails at the tasks will also be turned to stone.

It is not the first time we have encountered such going-to-sleep experiences. In earlier times one could still experience the passing over into sleep as the soul slipping out of its bodily sheath. The enchanted castle is an imagination of the moment of going to sleep when the soul, already loosened from the body, looks back upon it. The etheric formative forces, which have formed the human head and condensed it out of cosmic life, appear as a castle with many pillars and chambers. Enchanted within the hard skull-formation of the human body these mighty structures appear deathly silent and stoney.

With the help of an elemental being — the little grey man — the human consciousness, which would otherwise fall asleep at the moment of separation from the body, gains the strength to keep itself awake in a supersensory manner. Then it is shown what it must achieve in order not to be turned to stone. The three tasks inscribed on the tablet contain the hidden secret of a supersensory awakening of consciousness.

Human soul-life, though it appears as a unity, depends on the working together of three soul-forces. These forces, each of which has its own independent life, bear their impulses out of hidden spirit-worlds into our innermost being. All healthy experience we owe in the first instance to the instinctive harmony between these soul-members. Rudolf Steiner called them the sentient soul, intellectual soul and consciousness soul. In his Mystery Plays they appear in the form of Philia, Astrid and Luna. In Goethe's fairy-tale of the "Green Snake and the Beautiful Lily" they are portrayed as the three maids of the Beautiful Lily. The first of these soul-forces preserves in us the life of past times when the human soul, rich in feeling, still lived and moved in union with the powers of nature. The second has led us from a clairvoyant experience of the world to a comprehension of the natural and the human worlds; it has awakened our inner world with its ideas and deepened feelings. The third urges us to unfold our consciousness of personality. Everything which leads to independence of perception and action, and thus develops a free consciousness of self, we owe to this force which points the path to the future. Our unified consciousness is formed out of the harmony of these three soul forces. All three have a part to play in us but only by letting one's inner striving be guided by the consciousness soul can one unite with the future forces of the world. Such a man treads a moral path, directed by self-conscious responsibility, towards the supersensory. Considerable certainty of judgment is needed while penetrating the spiritual world if a person is not to fall prey to atavistic faculties of the soul which make the human being unfree on the path of the spirit. The consciousness soul alone, even though a nascent force, leads in our time to marriage with the higher self.

A heightened awareness of self is needed to perceive these three secretly active soul members. One does not penetrate to one's true inner world by psychologically dismembering oneself. It is of no use in moods of complacency or contrition to contemplate incessantly one's gifts or failings. In order to look at these formative soul-forces, which weave creatively behind the ebb and flow of perception, the sequence of ideas and the shreds of memories in our inner life, we need a key. And we find it only at the stage of imaginative cognition. Imaginative cognition does not mould the soul with inward brooding, but through actively living with the phenomena of blossoming and decaying: the nature forces of coming-into-being and passing away. The overcoming of fixed ideas by connecting with the realm of flowing pictures, which is formatively active within the world of appearances, also leads to a perception of objective soul-forces which create our inner life.

Anyone who wishes to grasp the supersensory life in world processes must first learn to carefully observe the phenomena of the world. An organizing mind, which knows how to bring together the profusion of perceptions in such a way that they illuminate one another and reveal their meaning to the observer, is the healthy preliminary stage. From looking correctly at the phenomena of the world there grows in the human spirit a comprehension of his own being.

Three tests, says the fairy-tale, are set the three brothers. The first consists of finding the king's daughter's thousand scattered pearls. It must be done by sundown — in waking consciousness. The two elder brothers do not succeed even with this first task and are turned to stone. Blockhead, however, is helped to find the pearls by the king of the ants and his army. The second task is to recover the key to the king's daughter's bedroom from the lake. It is accomplished with the help of the ducks. The third and hardest task is to identify the youngest and most lovely of the king's daughters while they are asleep. They look completely alike and can be told apart only because before going to sleep one had eaten a piece of sugar, the second some syrup and the third a spoonful of honey. Choosing the right one is therefore a matter of "taste". The queen bee of the beehive spared by Blockhead tastes the sleepers' lips. Blockhead can then recognize the youngest princess and the spell is broken. Everything is brought back to life; Blockhead marries the youngest sister and inherits the kingdom.

"Nature is an enchanted city turned to stone," says Novalis in his *Fragments*. Everywhere in the forms and phenomena of nature, creative spirit is trapped. Nature's development seems to have come to a halt, but through the continuing development of the human soul the world can be led towards its disenchantment. To develop, the human soul must not only look within itself but must become fructified by the wisdom-filled content of the world. This is fundamentally its eternal possession; it is only a matter of discovering it. In order to do so, however, the soul must extend its powers of perception. In the realm of the ants we can observe the activity of the senses and the will which unites them in a common task. The group-souls in the animal kingdom still possess great instinctive faculties which the human spirit must rediscover if it is to develop higher powers of soul.

Consider the duck: light and graceful on the water but an inelegant creature on land. On the ground the duck looks helpless; in the watery element it shows the skill of a diver. In this picture we can see possibilities for soul development. Often the animals set us an example in their earthly form of what we should attain in a spiritual way. Thus our moral thinking must learn to overcome its "fear of the water". A striving for knowledge demands that we should leave the firm ground of sense-experience in order to dive down into the flood of imaginative cognition. This is what opens the inner realm of the soul. It is now a matter of making the right choice, of turning towards the consciousness soul, the bearer of the future.

In fairy-tales, the image of the bee points towards an awakening of the most light-filled powers of consciousness. The bee's organic nature ordains that it produce honey. Similarly, man is created to transform into a special force everything earthly that he takes into himself. Bees know how to entice the noblest food from nature and transform it into sunlike honey. Man is able to do a similar thing on a spiritual plane: he can transform everything which he takes from the sense-world into the shining food of the spirit. But in order to do so he must awake in his inner nature of light. There was a stage in the old mysteries at which the initiate received the name of "bee". For such a man everything he met could become a chalice, out of which to drink nourishment for the soul.

The Egyptians represented their gods with animal heads: Horus appears with a hawk's head; the goddess of the magic of love, Bast, is shown with a cat's head.

The Egyptians felt that in the instincts there lived a more comprehensive wisdom than the knowledge man can acquire through his head. The human soul must first seek the guidance of these instincts before it can attain a knowledge higher than any purely rational thinking can provide. So in the "Miller's Drudge and the Cat", a cat appears to the poor miller's boy and takes him into her service for seven years. He has to follow her into the enchanted palace and live entirely with cats. She gives him silver tools and timber for him to make her a little silver house.

Everything that stands beneath the magic of moonlight appears to the clairvoyant as silver. Our dream consciousness (like all instinctive cleverness) is permeated with moon forces. This consciousness does not have its seat in the cerebrum, the forebrain, but is founded on a greater activity of the forces of the back of the brain. These forces played a much greater part in earlier ages than they do now. The strong development of the front part of the brain which promotes human intellect, focused on earthly things, has gradually repressed that other consciousness which was more subject to the effects of the moon. Hans, the miller's boy who has not developed fully the power of earthly understanding, is regarded as an idiot but he has not lost the ability to find the enchanted palace. The repressed powers of wisdom in the dream-nature are developed in Hans to a high degree.

At first it is still instinctive urges which take possession of this dim layer of consciousness so the human being can easily lose his freedom if he surrenders blindly to them. In the fairy-tale they take the form of cats. Hans allows himself to be taught by the cat without surrendering his own free will. "I don't dance with pussycats," he says when she asks him to dance with her. And so he remains free and she appears as a

splendid princess as soon as he has sufficiently transformed the moon forces in the hidden regions of his
soul: when he has built the silver house. Out of this dim
dream-consciousness a higher spiritual consciousness,
imaginative cognition, can be derived. That is the
reward of "seven years" faithful service.

In the "Golden Bird" the fox appears as the clever
adviser. He is not shown as a particularly noble force
but the seeker after the spirit cannot do without him.
Anyone seeking the golden bird, the golden horse and
the princess of the golden palace can easily lose the
firm ground of reality. He needs sound judgment
which he must get from the earth if he is not to waft
about in the spirit. Once he has reached his goal he can
learn to transcend this power of judgment which
guides him in an instinctive way. That is why the fox
demands that the king's son should cut off its head and
paws. Decapitation signifies the transformation of
egotistic forces which must become impersonal in
order to be spiritualized. In the *Chemical Wedding of
Christian Rosenkreuz,* a seventeenth-century work por-
traying the way into the supersensory, the beheading
of the king is a decisive event. The ability to assert
oneself at the right moment, presence of mind in
deciding and acting, is an egotistic instinct which we
develop on earth. Once it has become ennobled in the
service of spiritual endeavour it can shed its lower
nature. The fairy-tale recounts how the beheaded fox
turns out to be the beautiful princess's brother. He
becomes a royal power himself and stands in the
service of the spirit in man.

Towards the end of the Middle Ages the leaders
who gave spiritual direction to Western culture saw
clearly that man's consciousness was changing. Those

who understand the transformations human soul-forces undergo know that all holy traditions are doomed to extinction. The primal religious lore and practice with its symbolic language derive from experience of a higher world. When the inspired consciousness out of which they arose no longer stands behind them to infuse them with life, they lose their power. Man's ability to perceive the spiritual, to hear the divine Word, has faded. The human soul has forgotten the true "names of things"; language has become only a means of intellectual understanding.

There were circles of people resolved to regain a direct experience of the spirit for mankind. They spoke of the quest for the "lost Word" and worked to recover an inspired experience of the world. But they knew that mankind's powers of reason would not alone be able to find contact again with the creative spirit. What was needed were childlike soul qualities to rejuvenate and permeate man's whole being. It was felt that three virtues needed to flow into the ageing human consciousness: soul courage, to investigate the unexplored depths of the soul; compassion, to respond generously to the needs of the world; and open-mindedness, leading to an appreciation of the presence of the spirit. Judged coldly, these virtues can be seen like foolishness but they are "wisdom before God", as St Paul says. But the fairy-tales have their own way of arguing their case. The "Three Languages" tells of a boy who was stupid and could not learn anything. Untapped powers of mind and will slumber in the boy, but his father has no sympathy wishing only to "get something into the boy's head". Here we meet that simple-mindedness typified by Perceval which enfolds purity within it. For three years running the father sends his son to famous masters to have him educated. To his father's disgust all he learns is the language of dogs, birds and frogs. The father disowns the son who becomes a wanderer.

The wanderer's first task shows us that he is a seeker after the spirit who, having started on the path of higher knowledge, now finds himself on the threshold of new times. In *Faust,* Goethe depicts just such a figure. Faust can no longer unite his soul with the holy traditions. The Easter tidings, "the heavenly notes that seek him in the dust", no longer reach his heart, and so he turns to the earthly powers. A dog follows him into his quiet cell and prevents his soul from contemplation. Faust no longer understands St John's Gospel, for the dog's barking drowns all that would arise in his soul. The underworld, with its hellish din, drives away the voices of tranquillity.

In the "Three Languages", the boy seeks shelter at a castle. He is offered a dungeon filled with wild dogs that need appeasing with human sacrifices. The youth goes down without fear for he understands the language of dogs. The dogs tell him of a great treasure buried in the dungeon. The dogs guard it and are under a spell until it is dug up. The lord of the castle promises to make the youth his heir if he can accomplish the deed. The youth brings up the treasure and the barking dogs are silenced.

The dog is the guardian of the mysteries of the underworld: one of the twelve tasks of Hercules was to bring the hellhound up from the depths. Anyone who seeks the precious powers which slumber deep in the earth will meet the wild destructive forces that rule there and anyone who explores the world of the senses will come into contact also with the subhuman. Man has come very close to this realm for our technical knowledge works with underground forces. We can see how our humanity is consumed as we work with these material forces: the dogs demand human sacrifice, says the fairy-tale. Only someone who is initiated into the hidden language of nature can explore unscathed its depths and win from it the golden treasure. Enchanted world-will waits for a creative man. To master the gold by casting it into wisdom-filled forms is to possess it.

By developing a single sense — albeit at the cost of the harmony of the whole — animals have an advantage over human beings. With the dog it is as if its whole intelligence is poured into its nose. The dog can scent the fine emanations of a human trail and sniff out the bad intentions of someone creeping round a house. By his whole nature he is a detective. If a person has a propensity for recognizing the lower motives in people's actions, so that all human activity appears to him as all too human or basically selfish, we call him a cynic. The word is derived from the Greek for dog and means a dog's way of thinking. The Greek school of the cynics practiced this outlook, and the same tendency can be found in Freudian psychoanalysis which attributes all idealistic motivations (in art, religion and cognition) to repressed or sublimated animal urges. It discovers in the noblest of human beings the sub-human. This attitude has some justification, but where the seeker after knowledge admits no other then he sinks to the level of the dog. His whole wisdom is reduced to a sublimated sense of smell. *"Cave canem!"* stood at the gates of the ancient sanctuaries of wisdom: beware lest you fall victim to the dog in thee when you begin to recognize certain despicable forces as you stand on the threshold of hidden worlds! Hold fast always to reverence for the divine image of man.

The youth in the fairy-tale, having experienced the depths now seeks the heights. He travels to Rome, for in the language of the Middle Ages Rome represented the guardian of the most ancient holy traditions. When it was a question of the eternal in the human being, a question of the "soul's weal" about which the earth's depths could tell nothing, people turned to the Church. The fairy-tale is set at a turning-point in history. The chain of religious traditions is threatening to break. What is needed is a "miracle from above", a new injection from divine worlds if Christianity is to find its path. In spite of being clothed in the language of the Middle Ages, the pictures enable us to enter the world-historical nature of the situation. The youth passes a marsh where frogs are croaking. He understands their language and their message makes him thoughtful and sad. In Rome the Pope has died and the cardinals cannot agree on a successor. They beg God for a miraculous sign by which they will recognize the true successor. Meanwhile the youth enters the church where the cardinals are assembled and two white doves land on his shoulders. This is obviously the miraculous sign and the youth is made Pope. Then he has to celebrate mass but he does not know the words. Only by trusting in the immediate presence of the Holy Spirit can the youth dare to step up to the altar and celebrate the mass. The doves on his shoulders whisper rune-wise the divine words into his ear. But we have a presentiment that it is a different service, a new one sprung from the Spirit, which sounds from his lips.

With incredible audacity and great wisdom the fairy-tale speaks of the approach of a turning-point. An epoch of inspiration is about to begin and the sacred altar-service of Christianity is to be renewed. The youth chosen by the spirit no longer performs the office through the forces of tradition. The words of the ritual stream to him from immediate spirit-revelation. He finds the grace of the heights because he has attained and harnessed the power of the

depths. In the words and symbolism of the sacrifice of
the mass the language of heaven once lived. The
human word could become a messenger of the highest
divine deed, illuminating all earth existence. Bread
and wine, gifts of the earth, could be taken up by the
spirit and hallowed; things of earth began to speak of
their inner life.

This power of the spirit-word has died and can only
be renewed by someone who understands the language of the birds. When innocent senses begin to
unfold in the soul, the Word of the spheres can again
resound in words of earth. From where all creatures
reveal their being in musical tones the new power of
language flows to the man who can understand it. On
his way to the "lost word", this pilgrim of the spirit has
learned to read the signs of the times. For only out of a
recognition of the demands of the times can he gain
the courage for a new beginning. He has seen pro-
phetically how the traditional is coming to an end and
the new is clamouring to be formed. He understands
"what the frogs are croaking". Like a stringed instru-
ment on which the forces of the surroundings play, the
frog lives in and reacts to the changes of the weather
and atmospheric pressure. The frog dreams the
processes of the earth-soul: the movement of the air
and the rising and falling of the waters. Anyone who
has awakened the capacity to feel at one with nature's
flowering and fading can also become aware of the
needs and demands that arise in the evolution of
mankind. He learns to "know through compassion".
The weather signs of history reveal themselves to him:
"the frogs croak." He is dismayed by what he perceives
but his readiness to receive the spirit awakens all the
more strongly in his soul allowing him to bear the
inspiration of the heights down to the altar of the
earth.

11

Enchantment
and release

Goethe was well acquainted with the condition of slight
rapture in which the soul has a feeling of going out
beyond itself. He describes how this state of consciousness can rise to prophetic vision: "We all walk amid
mysteries. We are surrounded by an atmosphere in
which we do not know at all what is going on or how it is
linked to our destinies. So much is certain, however,
that under special circumstances the sensitive feelers
of our souls can reach beyond the limits of the body,
and the soul is granted a presentiment, indeed a real
view of the future."

In the "Three Languages" we find the frogs bearing
this "atmospheric consciousness". The frog exhibits an
intermediate stage in the organic evolution of species:
between gill and lung breathers. Unable to experience
the totality of fish existence, the frog seems to be
constantly dreaming of a lost world. We can feel
something deeply melancholic in the frog's nature,
perhaps sharing with him a similar experience for man
also has had to pass through many forms before
attaining his upright stance. These stages also dream
in us, in deeply sunken layers of consciousness that can
break through under unusual conditions: when a
loosening of the etheric forces from the physical body
occurs these primal experiences can make themselves
felt again.

By placing the "Frog King" (also known as the "Frog Prince" or "Iron Heinrich") at the beginning of their collection, the Grimms showed a remarkable feeling for the essential nature of the fairy-tale experience. This begins with memory pictures or even only memory feelings rising up, coming as it were from the depths of a well.

Melancholy comes over the soul when in its depths a memory stirs which reminds it of ancient modes of consciousness when the living gold of wisdom played into its feelings. Once it was rich, graced with the might of the sun, for it belonged to a cosmos in which the Fall had not yet worked as a darkening power. In the "Frog King", the king's daughter weeps by the well into which her golden ball has fallen. Grief for the lost wisdom of the sun is the beginning of a slight memory in which the return of the golden age is heralded. In the seeking soul a consciousness stirs that can dive down into the depths of the soul to bring up shining pictures from our slumbering cosmic memory. Watching running water can lead to a slight entrancement that brings clairvoyance, so people who live close to water — especially children who love the water element above all — are more prone to a loosening of the soul than those firmly rooted on dry land. In many myths and legends we see a water being enticing children into the water. In the past kelpies and nixies were visible to clairvoyance. Everyone has something of the watery nature in him as a memory of a former stage of man's evolution.

But the soul can again grow beyond the narrow confines of sense-consciousness. The waterman consciousness is trying to return from the depths of dreams, at first as a dim figure, and, when not lit by understanding, thrusting itself forward like a nightmare. The soul must become familiar with it and learn, even though at first unwillingly, to hold a dialogue with it as with a second self.

In the fairy-tale, the frog in the well asks the princess why she cries. The princess tells him and he offers to retrieve the golden ball if she will love him and let him live with her. The princess agrees thinking that the frog cannot escape the well and her ball is retrieved. The princess, having forgotten the frog, is startled and frightened when he appears the next day asking her to fulfil her promise. Her father, the wise old king, tells her she must keep her promise and she reluctantly assists the frog to eat from her golden plate. But revolted and angry, only her father's command will induce her to take the frog to her bedroom. As she lies in bed the frog crawls to her and demands to be taken into her bed. She picks him up and angrily throws him against the wall whereupon he changes into a handsome prince.

It requires a considerable strengthening of the will to awaken the hidden self that lies enchanted in the weaving of dreams. The soul's initiative must be at work to wrest it from its disguise; only then does it appear in its true spiritual form. That is the awakening of the supersensory man who comes from primal times and brings cosmic memory into the present. A dream-like, backward-looking life is set free and can bend its vision forwards: a "prophetic" spiritual power that points to the future is born.

The fairy-tale also touches on an initiation of the heart through the figure of faithful Hans. While the prince is bewitched, his servant Hans has fastened iron bands around his heart to keep it from bursting with grief. A man who seeks the spirit and loyally follows the mystical path is the servant of the hidden spirit-man and knows he must place all his powers in the service of the awakening of the immortal part of his being. Only through a deep calmness of the heart, wherein all the urging and wishing of the earthly man are silenced, will it be possible for him to follow this path to the end. The heart must be held in "iron bands". But the heart-forces which have gone through death begin to celebrate their resurrection as soon as the soul, married to the spirit, enters the spirit's kingdom.

The meeting with the powers of the heart and the mystery of their transformation is often represented by the imagination of a lion. We have already encountered this picture in the "Water of Life" and in the "Twelve Huntsmen": first the threatening lion, then the wise lion. On the way to initiation, a person who is to awake to the spirit may behold the interior of his own body. When he rises with his soul out of the bodily sheath on falling asleep, the separate organs of his body can begin to reveal their nature. He becomes aware that every organ has a predisposition to create an animal form. The heart hides a courageous, proud lion. But the lion has another side: an urge to violence and power. In the lungs lives an eagle that longs to rise above the heaviness of earth but is forcefully restrained by the laws of the body.

When the heart and lungs play into each other, the griffin, a lion-eagle, appears to spiritual sight. Such fabulous creatures, known from mythology, have not sprung from an extravagant fantasy but from an ancient dreamlike vision which saw in the griffin an image of the powers of wisdom united with audacity tempting man to tear himself away from the dullness of earth. The griffin bears the desire for light which Lucifer has implanted in us, giving wings to the imagination and spirit-vision to the soul.

Initiation into the heart-powers demands courage and an acceptance of destiny. Everything that lives in the soul's depths as indignation against the forces of destiny, as arrogance or wounded pride, is reflected in imaginative pictures (or even in dreams). "The lion must become a lamb," was said to indicate the will to conciliation which is ready to take destiny upon itself. But in the highest sense this points to the power of sacrifice of the one who would take upon himself the guilt of the whole earth. In the human heart, when a force begins to be liberated by dispelling despondency and accepting destiny, there appears the picture of a bird that flies up rejoicing. It means that the liberating forces are beginning to work in the heart. And the bird that longs to fly in thanksgiving, lilting and leaping free from the dust of earth, is the lark.

A deep connection between the lark and the lion forces is found in the fairy-tale of the "Leaping, Lilting Lark". A man about to go on a long journey asks his three daughters what he should bring them. The eldest wishes for pearls; the second for diamonds; the youngest, his favourite, asks for "a lilting, leaping lark". On his way home he finds a lark in a tree but when he sets his servant to fetch it a roaring lion springs out threatening to eat anyone who dares to steal his bird. The man can save himself only by promising to give the lion the first thing he meets on his return home. This happens to be his youngest daughter. He gives her the lark and tells her that he has betrothed her to the lion. She accepts her destiny, bids farewell and is received by the lion with all his court, for he is a great king. By night he appears in human form, by day they sleep.

It is characteristic of the sentient soul that it should wish for pearls. Pearls represent dreaming wisdom. (Dante calls the moon the "eternal pearl in the sea of

heaven"). It is equally characteristic of the intellectual
soul that it loves diamonds: it seeks to understand the
world in cold, clear-cut ideas. But the youngest of the
soul forces, the consciousness soul, seeks more: in it,
the will to freedom is awakening. It seeks victory over
the heaviness of earth, and the awakening of an
immortal spirit-power that presses heavenward. To
travel this path requires daring and sacrifice but it
knows what is necessary to meet this spiritual goal.

We have mentioned how the animal forms underly-
ing the human organs can be perceived. To clairvoyant vision, however, the sleeping human figure
assumes a particular animal form. Rudolf Steiner
describes how the perception of this form reaches into
the day as personal motivation. "During the day I am
not aware of it; but it lives in me as a conflux of forces
... which drag me down and tempt me to succumb to
personal interests. And when we develop this impression more and more we come to recognize the reality
of Lucifer and the part he plays in our evolution. The
further we look back clairvoyantly to the time that
corresponds to the Paradise Imagination, the more
beautiful becomes the structure which only at a later
time really recalls our animal nature. And if, further-
more, we go back to the Paradise epoch, we may then
say that these forms ... [of bull, lion, and eagle] may
also be for us in a certain sense, symbols of beauty."
And even further back Lucifer appears in sublime
beauty to the spirit's vision. His form is then revealed,
for he is "On the one hand the Spirit of Beauty, and on
the other hand, the Spirit of egoism." And it is this
spirit in whose company we are from going to sleep
until waking: "The moment the veil is lifted we ... find
that Lucifer is at our side ... man is moving towards a
future when every time he awakens, he will have the
impression, at first like a fleeting dream, but subse-

quently ever more clearly, that his companion during the night was Lucifer."*

This fact was fully known to the Greeks as an initiation-experience and they called this figure Eros. Eros, who awakes in the soul a love of what is beautiful and great but at the same time fills the soul with egotistic feelings, they depicted as mediator between men and gods. Eros will not rest until Psyche — the human soul he loves passionately — is carried up to Olympus. The ancient fairy-tale of "Eros (or Amor) and Psyche", reflects this mystery. It is important to note the relationship of this motif to the "Lilting, Leaping Lark", a relationship which Wilhelm Grimm also pointed out in his comments. He says, comparing the two: "The heart is tested, and all earthly and evil falls away before the knowledge born of pure love. Our story agrees that light brings misfortune and night, which unchains all bonds, releases the magic spell." What Grimm calls misfortune seems so only to earthly judgment. Psyche enjoys the love of her husband without ever having seen him. They belong to each other only in the kingdom of the night. Her sisters try to persuade her that he is a beastlike monster and provoke her into lighting the lamp. But the lamp reveals the god of love in all his beauty, and as she gazes on him a drop of burning oil falls on his right shoulder and wakes him. He rises in the air without a word. Psyche must undergo many trials for the sake of her lost husband.

This is a pictorial description of the trials and purifications which are set before the soul on the path to immortal life. They begin straight after that nocturnal discovery. It is the lamp of cognition which Psyche lights, though her desire for knowledge is unpurified

* Rudolf Steiner, *The Effects of Spiritual Development*, London 1978, pp. 132f, 133, 134–36.

and filled with scepticism. What in the kingdom of night is a sublime figure of beauty, which however must be hidden from the soul's view, can become filled with passion when the soul passes from waking to sleeping or from sleeping to waking, and so can appear in tremendous animal forms. Before the daytime consciousness a sphinxlike figure stands like a memory picture: the monster which Psyche's sisters mention. In a certain sense it is also a lion figure which remains as an imaginative manifestation for our daytime consciousness. The powers of the heart which are to be transformed and set free appear as the picture of the kingly lion. In the kingdom of the night it is a sublime figure, companion of the soul.

The "Lilting, Leaping Lark" tells how the lion avoids candlelight. When in spite of every precaution the light from a torch falls on him he becomes a white dove. Before flying away the dove tells the youngest daughter that he must fly away into the world but will let fall drops of red blood and white feathers to allow her to follow and release him from the spell.

As in "Eros and Psyche" it is the torch of cognition which casts a ray upon the mystery hidden in the depths of night. Now the dove shows the path which has to be followed: it is the mystic path of seven stages. In the "Twelve Brothers" we have already met those "seven years" which are necessary for the release. The Holy Spirit becomes the guide upon this way. But the fairy-tale picture indicates that it is not only the power of the spirit which gives the soul its direction. At every seventh step the dove lets fall not only a white feather but also a drop of red blood. The soul steps forth upon her way still under the influence of blood-love. Eros is still the winged power of her heart; he has only been partly spiritualized. When the seven years have nearly come to an end and the wife's hopes rise, she loses the trail. That again appears to be a misfortune but it is a sign that the soul has been given its freedom. It does not need guidance but must learn to act from its inmost freedom. She asks the sun and the moon and the four winds for news of the dove. Only the south wind knows; but the sun and the moon give her useful gifts: a little box and an egg. The soul has become capable of experiencing itself in the cosmos; on the path of cognition it has outgrown its narrow earth consciousness. She must now overcome the lower nature. She must experience the "inner south". The south wind tells her that the dove has become a lion and is fighting with a dragon by the Red Sea; the dragon however is an enchanted princess. The "night wind" imparts to the soul the thought powers to vanquish the passion nature. The heart that is to be freed from the might of the blood needs the wisdom of the head, for the heart alone would never come through the battle of the "Red Sea". When, however, the lion and the dragon have regained their human shape the dragon princess carries the lion king to her kingdom on a griffin. The wife is left to find the palace in which the two are living. She is told that the wedding is being prepared. The gift of the sun is a beautiful dress which she trades with the dragon princess for a night with the bridegroom. Drugged, the lion king does not recognize his true wife as she sits by his bed and tells him of her seven-year pilgrimage: to him it is only as if the wind were rustling in the trees. The gift of the moon, a hen with twelve golden chicks, is also traded for a night with the bridegroom but this time he pours away the sleeping draught having been fore-warned by his servant. He recognizes his faithful wife and they fly home on the griffin to find their child grown up and most beautiful.

In these pictures are hidden the inner experiences

of the seeker after the spirit. Once the mystic on his path has learnt to control the lower nature, has tamed the dragon and freed it from its enchantment, he has to find the power to rise above the confines of the senses to the spirit. In Middle Ages mysticism, the griffin stood for the supersensory divine vision. Dante represents Christ in this form (*Purgatory*, can. 20 & 31). He teaches that the twin nature of the redeemer is revealed in the eagle and the lion: the more divine aspect of his being in the eagle and the more human aspect in the lion. These two aspects are constantly interchanging but in the deepest sense are changeless. In him earthly and heavenly forces are held in balance. Christ holds the balance within the soul but this does not contradict what we have already said about the griffin being the picture of the enthusiastic Luciferic powers. Christ as the "mystic griffin" stands as the true "Lucifer", the true light-bringer who will bring the true spirit-light instead of the deceptive one. Only when the ethical and sensual man are brought into harmony can the liberation of the human heart be effected.

But here watchfulness is necessary. Many mystics bore only a refined sensuality into the spirit realms thinking they had tamed their passions with asceticism but the erotic colouring of many mystical visions and the dark fervour of many hymns to the Madonna and to Christ suggest otherwise. The dragon princess flies away on the griffin and gives the lion-king a magic draught. In such cases the sense-nature is "sublimated" and not really transformed. The true spiritual light is kept hidden from the mystic by illusion in his soul. The lower urges, which would appear to be spiritual, must first be attracted by the radiance of the purified soul-forces and overcome. But the soul which has travelled the path of purification has been permeated with cosmic powers of light and appears now in the sun-besparkled dress. The mystery of a new spirit-body has been revealed to her with rejuvenated, lighter senses ready to unfold; she can open the egg and release the golden chicks. The sensual nature of man, on coming into contact with these supersensory gifts which the soul was able to acquire from cosmic heights, loses its power. The spirit-consciousness finally becomes free from the lower urges which held it in illusion. Now it can harvest the experience which the soul has acquired on her mystic pilgrimage. Eros becomes transfigured. The griffin bears the lovers away from the Red Sea. The lion is transformed into the pure shape of man.

In the fairy-tale, as soon as a force has been freed from instinctual life and enters the sphere of waking cognition it appears in human form. It has been freed from enchantment. The deepest mystical process which can take place in the depths of the soul is the spiritualization of Eros: by degrees the might of Lucifer is transformed into the light of the Holy Spirit.

The fairy-tale "Jorinda and Joringel", with its picture of the blood-red flower holding a sparkling dewdrop, points to the hallowing of the forces of the blood. The flower has the power to release from enchantment and Joringel uses it to free Jorinda who has been turned into a nightingale.

The lark and the nightingale can be seen as opposites. The lark sings early in the morning a song of rejoicing, of thanksgiving, while the nightingale sings its sad song in the evening. In the lark the liberated heart forces resound, but the nightingale sings of unredeemed longings. Oppressed by fear of earth, the nightingale longs to free itself from the confines of earth.

131

The nightingale stands under the power of the moon: Jorinda is bewitched in the moonlight. And it is the moon which makes the soul mournful and full of yearning, for it casts a spell over the soul. In the Apocalypse of St John there is the image of a woman clothed in the sun holding the moon beneath her feet. Human blood stands under the spell of the moon and cannot by itself gain freedom. It needs the power of grace from above, falling like heaven's dew into earthly feeling and wishing. The motif of the red flower holding a pearl of dew points to the mystery of the Grail and the redemptive quality of the blood of Christ. Only the Christ can heal the deep melancholy that comes when existence is felt as suffering. There is only one magic flower which can release the nightingale from the spell.

Goethe's friend Jung-Stilling wove this fairy-tale into his childhood recollections. It is him we have to thank for its survival. It was told to him by an aunt as they sat in a forest clearing, while old father Stilling went to look for wood. The magical forces weaving in the woods woke higher senses in the old man and he had visions of those who had died leading exalted lives and of fairy-tale palaces which beckoned him to enter. And so, while the young folk were immersed in the fairy-tale, the old man was living in those regions where fairy-tales really happen.

12

The powers of darkness

Novalis said that the truly moral man is also a poet. For him poetry was a revelation of the moral sense to which knowledge of a future world order is entrusted. When this moral organ awakens and becomes creative, it becomes aware of its limits, for the laws of nature disregard its demands. The idealist's will to act is condemned to impotence by those very laws and he must painfully realize that he stands before the world with his hands bound.

The fairy-tale of the "Girl Without Hands" deals with this question of the moral sense condemned to impotence. The story tells how the devil promises a poor miller wealth if he will give him what is standing behind his mill. The miller accepts the condition, thinking that it could only be an apple-tree but it is the miller's daughter that the devil has in mind. But the girl is so pious and pure that the devil fails to gain power over her. He manages, however, to make the miller cut off his daughter's hands but he cannot touch her soul. The human being who has lost the fullness of the ancient wisdom — who has become "poor" — makes a pact with a power whose aims are at first inscrutable. Goethe represents this power which rises out of the darkness of the earth as Mephistopheles. He is not the tempter from the Garden of Eden: that is

Lucifer who works in our desires and is the power who originally forced us into incarnation. Lucifer casts the human soul under "enchantment", but is not yet its destroyer. The fairy-tale indicates the difference in a picture. The miller thinks of the apple tree behind the mill. This is actually the Tree of Knowledge, which the serpent took possession of. But the devil seeks to win over the soul's powers that have remained pure and virginal and so destroy the eternal in the human being.

At the end of the Middle Ages the ancient knowledge began to die away while new intellectual powers emerged promising mankind new knowledge of the world. It was then that men began to feel this sinister and still inscrutable power. Research into the world of the senses by means of purely earthly laws and the mastery of this world through technology are the gifts that come from this pact with the devil, described in anthroposophy and Persian mythology as Ahriman, and as Mephistopheles in Faust. The fairy-tales of "Bearskin" and the "Devil's Grimy Brother" describe the same power that promises riches but threatens to cast darkness over the depths of the moral sense, and to deliver all human endeavour to the earthly and the transient.

In each of the fairy-tales the devil harvests the soul after a certain time. By giving herself over to purely intellectual knowledge the soul allows its bond with the divine to gradually die and comes within the devil's realm. The miller's daughter, however, spends this period in fear of God and without sin, and when the devil approaches, draws a chalk circle round herself. The devil cannot reach these powers of soul guarded in purity; the magic circle of the white powers protects the virgin. In the pursuit of materialistic knowledge, man can be trapped by a black magic that can destroy the soul, but there are ways of purification, or "white

magic", that can be set against it. The fairy-tale shows
how a human being may devote himself without harm
to the earth-knowledge that binds him to the
Ahrimanic power as long as he can see through this
power and at the same time develop and strengthen
his moral sense. The virgin is saved, but she has to
sacrifice her hands. The higher man becomes lamed in
his will. He can still form thoughts of the divine but can
no longer realize them.

The maiden then sets out on her pilgrimage. In the
moonlight she finds a royal orchard. Under the
protection of an angel she enters the garden and eats a
pear. When first man ate from the Tree of Knowledge,
he was driven out and exiled from paradise lest he
should eat from the Tree of Life. While knowledge is
associated with the apple, the other tree which has
remained untouched can be seen as the pear tree. The
apple, with its firm substance and round form, was
always felt to be the fruit by which man becomes
conscious of his own being and grasps himself as an
independent self. The form of the pear and its ability
to readily dissolve into liquid provides a contrast to the
apple. A dreamlike wisdom, not wide-awake cognition, is the fruit that ripens on the pear tree. Here a
world opens that should be protected from the
earthly-egotistic consciousness. It is angel wisdom into
whose realm the soul may enter only at night. In this
realm she becomes a queen, and the king, who loves
her because she is so beautiful and pious, has silver
hands made for her. The soul that is permitted to wake
in magical moonlight and enter hidden worlds may
also receive "silver hands". The kingdom of the night
makes the senses fruitful; it wakes the imagination
which can rise above earth-reason and comprehend by
artistic creativity a world which is still hidden from
sight.

But the devil interferes and the young queen is banished from court. In a materialistic age the soul that has awakened to higher life finds that its experience of the spirit is slandered and rejected by the world. But only in loneliness of soul, thrust back upon itself, does the inner man find true freedom. The higher self begins to grow strong precisely when it experiences the opposition in which our eternal being stands to earth-reality, a reality which the Ahrimanic spirit first teaches us to grasp in its entirety. Only then does the higher self discover the holy place within the soul where the laws of nature no longer prevail and freedom holds full sway.

The rejected queen lives for seven years in a little house, in front of which hangs a sign: "All are welcome." An angel cares for her and her little son, called Sorrowful. This fairy-tale points to a path of initiation of the soul. Very significant is the meeting in the lonely house with the king who has searched for seven years. At first he does not recognize his wife, for she has grown new living hands. As tokens, however, the angel shows him the silver hands. The soul regains the full power to act once her forces can be directed in inner freedom. The spirit need no longer live only in fantasy for it now possesses the power of transformation. Instead of the silver hands, she has been given living ones: the evil spell is broken.

The experience of awakening inwardly to ourselves, just as we awaken outwardly by contact with the sense-world, is often depicted in fairy-tales. The tale of the "Glass Coffin", for example, tells of a series of acts of self-awakening.

A tailor lost in a wood climbs a tree to sleep. The wind is strong but he has his flat iron to hold him down. In the darkness he sees a light which he follows until he comes to a tiny house where he is lodged by a little old man. In the morning he witnesses a furious battle between a big black bull and a beautiful stag. The stag kills the bull and carries the tailor away. They stop at the foot of a cliff, the stag opens a hidden door with its antlers, and a voice from inside the rock invites the tailor into the secret kingdom of the rock.

Every evening the wind blows away the dried-up consciousness of intellectual man as he begins to loose himself from his body, for his consciousness lacks weight. If our conceptual life is not to be dissipated when we go to sleep, it will have to acquire inner weight. From the point of view of spiritual schooling it needs a strengthening of its thought powers to enable it to become conscious during sleep: the tailor carries his flat iron with him. The fairy-tale also graphically depicts how the human consciousness sleeps its way into the elemental world; how it is received by the consciousness of an elemental spirit and how it can wake up again. It experiences, from the outside as it were, the mighty battle that always takes place within the human organism whenever we wake up. Stag and bull struggle with each other.

These animals represent contrasts in formative forces. The bull's horns can be seen as a thickening of the skin: the powerful urges which surge up from below towards the head are caught, as it were, and dammed up in the horns. The stag's antlers are quite different: they are replaced every year and grow branch by branch. The stag's bones have become rejuvenating forces. The stag has rescued from the heaviness of the body a part of the formative forces of the skeleton and sent them up towards the light. Powers of resurrection reveal themselves above the skull-form of the stag, overcoming the death-forces working down from the head. This is why in legends the cross appears between the stag's antlers.

The upper nature of the human being brings us the powers of consciousness; every morning this upper nature has to renew its battle to push the actions of the metabolic system back into place for during sleep this system takes over the whole body. Only then can we wake up in our heads. But from the depths of the lower nature, which sends up nourishing forces and substances, all the lower urges stream up in sleep and darken the spirit-consciousness.

The fairy-tale sees these lower urges as the black bull, who is also a sinister magician. If with heightened powers of consciousness one can thrust these darkening forces out of the head one comes to a spiritual awakening before the physical morning awakening: one experiences the victory of the stag over the bull and the entry of the tailor into the secret kingdom behind the cliff.

Similarly, the castle of the Grail can be entered only in a mysterious way: it rises up in the evening before the seeker after the spirit. This is an experience of going to sleep, or rather of spiritual awakening while the body is falling asleep. The way in which the formative forces work in the body of the sleeper can reveal itself to imaginative vision. When the spirit does not go over into unconscious sleep, but manages consciously to look back upon the etheric body while it is going out from the physical body, certain quite definite pictures appear. Rudolf Steiner said: "As we approach our etheric body we feel as if we were approaching something which repels us. We come as it were to a spiritual rock. Later we feel as if we were admitted into something, as if we were now inside ..."*

* *The Effects of Spiritual Development*, London 1978, pp. 91f.

138

At these moments we become aware of the vegetative processes which replace the forces which have been used up during the day, and above all renew the substances used up in the brain. Then the brain appears not as the anatomist would see it, but as a castle in which the human being lies enchanted — forsaken by his consciousness. "Symbolized by the brain situated in the skull, terrestrial man appears like an enchanted being living in a castle. We see our human entity as if imprisoned behind castle walls. The symbol of this, the shrunken symbol as it were, is our skull ... And then from the rest of the organism there stream upwards the forces which sustain this being who is imprisoned in the skull as in a fortified castle." Rudolf Steiner goes on to describe how in the Legend of the Grail the sword and the bleeding lance are brought into the castle: the lance that gave the Grail King the wound that cannot be healed and appears to wound him again every evening. We know from Wolfram von Eschenbach's version of Perceval that this lance-thrust was given to the Grail King by a wicked magician.

In the "Glass Coffin", it is also a master of black magic who enters the castle and enchants the count and his sister. The tailor, who has entered the rock through an iron door, finds a glass case with a miniature castle inside and a glass coffin containing a beautiful maiden. The tailor succeeds in waking her and she tells him the story of her enchantment. Her brother was transformed into the stag and the black magician took the form of the black bull to fight against him. Through the victory over the bull everything can now be set free and restored, and the tailor can lead the awakened maiden to the altar.

In this fairy-tale it is not the mystery of the Grail that is placed before the soul, but the region in which it takes place. The etheric forces which have formed the brain and permeated it appear as the glass coffin in which a maiden, sunk in a death sleep, rests. The soul has frozen in its own intellectuality. But it is not death; she awaits the awakening. It is the same glass coffin in which Snow White rests after she has tasted the poisoned apple. The power of darkness, which climbs up from the depths of the body and poisons the fine organization of the brain, maims the spirit-consciousness: thus the higher intuitive faculties have been sent to sleep in the course of human evolution. But they can be set free once more by the victory over the "magician" and revitalized. The overcoming of materialism is more than an intellectual affair: it is an action of the will brought about by the self reaching down into hidden realms of the soul. It calls for a deed of awakening.

To perform this deed you must meet with the spiritual causes of that darkening of the soul. The magician or the witch in the fairy-tale must first be recognized, for in this recognition of the Evil One's activity a first awakening of the inner man takes place. There are teachers and parents troubled because the fairy- tales depict the wicked and the sinister in all their worldly power. These people are happy to tell of beautiful maidens and noble princes but would prefer not to mention the witches, wicked stepmothers and mighty magicians. But if we dilute the descriptions of the dark powers or leave them out altogether, we take from the fairy-tale its power of awakening, even though this power works unconsciously. For knowledge of evil calls up the power of the good in human hearts.

The way in which true fairy-tales wisely deal with light and darkness creates in the listener a healthy sense of reality. Anyone who is deeply immersed in the victory of the good powers, as is always represented and celebrated at the end of a fairy-tale, experiences evil as a necessity in the world. It is the power through which the good can first awaken to its own being. The human kingdom can shine out only against a background of darkness.

It is the same with all motifs which include an inexorable punishment of the wicked. Fundamentally they are apocalyptic imaginations: pictures of a last judgment which in the light of the spiritual world reveals itself as a self-judgment. The purifying working of the spirit, conquering illusion and destroying the transient, effects the liberation of the eternal kernel of man's being. So it is that many pronounce their own sentence: for example the haughty servant in the "Goose Girl". "White horses" are to drag her to death: the forces of wisdom, which have cleared themselves of all sense-darkness, cause the lower intelligence to feel its earth-heaviness; it feels itself gradually destroyed by them. In the fairy-tale of the "White Bride and the Black Bride" the same kind of thing happens to the old witch and her black daughter; there the wicked woman is so dazzled that she does not suspect anything when the question is put to her: "What does a woman deserve who has done thus and so?" She answers the question as if she were pronouncing judgment on another soul. In the soul-world which we enter after death we too shall find ourselves looking at our actions and attitudes objectively, and in the light of that higher world learning to judge them.

"Snow White" describes the inner restlessness that drives the wicked queen to the wedding feast. She is afraid, but goes nevertheless. She is forced by an inner urge to step into the red-hot slippers in which she dances to her death. In the "Juniper Tree" the inner nature of the last judgment is expressed. The consciousness of the guilty stepmother is transformed during the bird's song; at first she keeps her ears and eyes closed. But the roaring fills her ears and the lightning flashes before her eyes. The house seems to rock and burst into flames. The stepmother, conscious of her guilt, is driven by inner terror out of the house because she thinks the world must be coming to an end. Thus she brings on her fate to be crushed by the millstone.

Moral realities, which are at the same time the destruction and re-creation of the world, will in the future, and indeed already in earthly life, overcome the human soul. The domain of conscience, which has been more or less veiled from the soul, will break through more and more strongly. It will uplift and console, or oppress and destroy, for it can bring experiences that can only be compared in power with catastrophes in nature. Again the words of Novalis are apt here: "The true writer of fairy-tales is a seer of the future."

In Germanic apocalyptic imagery the giant wolf appears as the powers of darkness unchained. The image of the wolf indicates powers which by their nature do not stem from man's inward self, but have gained entry to him when he applied his will to the world of matter and began increasingly to renounce the gods' world of light.

In Persian lore, man as the servant of the powers of light was called upon at all times to fight against Ahriman who is the ossifying agency within the hidden formative forces of man's being. In every child the most tender formative forces are led into rigidity and in the course of adolescence the powers of imagination and fantasy are darkened and finally devoured by earthly desires. Very small children are especially fond of the story of the "Wolf and the Seven Young

Kids", because they can see something of their own destiny in its story. The urges of the child's soul are pure and as yet untouched by any darkness. But the school-age child opens out hungrily and not entirely innocently to the external world of the senses. The child wants to know about and experience everything but awakening to the earth-world brings with it a meeting with the darkening powers of matter. The wolf devours the young kids, says the fairy-tale, for they open the door to him because he knows how to disguise himself.

The deceptive power that knows how to mislead the unsuspecting feelings and aims to destroy the light-nature in man is always portrayed by a wolf. But why is it seven little kids? Wherever we meet the number seven in fairy-tales the action of the seven ancient planets is indicated. This planetary world implanted sevenfold soul-urges in man, just as the twelve senses stem from the twelvefold nature of the zodiac. Before we might receive the self, the germ of the immortal individuality, we were given the urges out of which the realm of feeling, the astral body, is built up. One expression of this law can be found in the musical scale with its seven notes. The sevenfold planetary forces are reflected as much in the higher abilities of the soul as in the lowest instincts. Hence the imaginations in the various fairy-tales and myths also vary. Thus we see seven ravens, seven dwarves, seven little kids and the seven-headed dragon. Ancient wisdom taught that the sevenfold planetary action formed seven main organs in the human body: brain, lungs, kidneys, heart, gall bladder, liver and spleen. In ancient medicine these organs were regarded as microcosmic representations of the Moon, Mercury, Venus, the Sun, Mars, Jupiter and Saturn. The sevenfold light-nature of the human soul, to which the "seven candlesticks" in religious symbolism correspond, can come to life in these seven organs. There is not only a head-consciousness; other organs also bear attitudes and thoughts, a kind of organ-consciousness. But the innocent, light-filled soul falls victim to the fate inherent in incarnation. As it is drawn into the material nature of the earth-body, the organ-consciousness is extinguished. It remains bound in the subconscious depths of our human nature.

Only the tenderest of the young kids escapes this fate. The little kid creeps into the clock case: the most childlike of all soul forces hides in the heart. There it still speaks, for the wolf has not been able to destroy it. It alone finds the "mother" again and can tell her what has happened to the others. Allied with the wisdom that has reawakened in the mother-depths of the soul, the unscathed heart-power can find again the other powers of the soul which have been obscured. The reawakening of the supersensory nature of man is portrayed in the happy release of the kids from the belly of the monster. The heavy material nature is in the process of becoming completely hardened. The powers of dead intellectual thinking, of egotistic feeling and blind willing, act like stones, dragging consciousness down into earth-heaviness. They weigh upon the lower bodily consciousness like a nightmare; but the spiritual nature with its organs of light can tear itself away from the death-sleep of matter.

The story of "Little Red Cap" (Little Red Riding Hood) is related to this. The young soul-power, recognizable by the red hood as the ego beginning to experience itself in the blood and to speak out of the blood, goes to visit the grandmother who represents the primal ancestor. "Little Red Cap" heralds a turning point in evolution. The soul, conscious of its self, loses itself in the attractions of the sense-world and the ancient spirit-consciousness forsakes her. She can no longer find the primal wisdom when she reaches down into her own depths: the wolf has seized the hidden formative forces within her. A darkness that would devour the young self as well threatens to break out from the depths of man's being. Rapacious greed, instead of a holy memory of the gods, dwells in these depths: the beast gazes at us from our own abyss.

A wakeful power of cognition, on the track of the wolf, is the only thing that can come to the rescue. In the fairy-tale it is the huntsman who finds the wolf and rescues Little Red Cap and the primal ancestor out of the stomach of the sleeping monster.

The child-force of the young self is waiting to be freed from the constraining embrace of the heavy earth-consciousness. This can no longer come about solely through the ancient traditions of wisdom. These traditions had themselves been obscured before the self lost its connection with the spiritual world. The primal ancestor is devoured and so Red Riding Hood is also devoured with her. For man, having lost the remembrance of his holy origin, loses in the end his true humanity as well. He is devoured by the animal.

The rescue of the human self from the death by suffocation which materialism threatens, brings a renewal of the true primal knowledge.

13

The Michael mystery

With earthly incarnation the human being enters a field of forces in which he has difficulty asserting himself in his true being. The power of darkness is too great for the soul's initial powers of resistance. It will be cursed and enchanted and swallowed by the dark power. Unsuspectingly overcome by blind urges, it enters the fatal circle. A miracle is necessary to allow the soul to break its bonds.

In the fairy-tales helpful beings, trials of endurance and deeds of sacrifice effect this liberation. But only very seldom is the countenance of that spirit-power revealed who can arm the human being with such strength that he can emerge as victor from the darkness.

St John describes the archetype of those battles fought for the eternal in man: the Archangel Michael fights in the heavens for the sun-arrayed, star-crowned virgin about to give birth. The great dragon with seven heads stands before her waiting to devour the new-born child.

All battles for the spirit fought on earth to wrest humanity from the powers of transience are reflections of this deed of Michael. Thus Perseus who frees Andromeda is the spiritual knight of the Greek world of saga, and Apollo who kills the python may be felt as the Greek Michael. St George who rescues the maiden from the dragon represents Michael in Christian legend.

Faced with the power of the dragon the archetype of man must be set up again. That is the mission of the Michael warrior. The folk tales too know such heroes who save the maiden. The motif appears most clearly in the fairy-tale of the "Two Brothers". One of the brothers, on climbing the dragon's mountain, finds a church. On the altar are three chalices and an inscription: "He who drains these goblets will become the strongest man on earth. He will wield the sword that lies buried outside the door." The youth finds the sword but cannot move it, so he drinks from the chalices. Now he is strong enough to draw the sword out of the earth and kill the seven-headed monster.

The sword that helps to conquer the dragon and the power to take possession of it are kept in a holy place. Human strength is not enough in such a battle: the dragon is stronger than any soul's power. Only from the altar can the individuality receive the highest strength. The three chalices show the spirit-seeker's need for a threefold assimilation of the Christ-forces: it is not enough to receive the healing forces only with the understanding or aspiration of the heart. The number three in fairy-tales and religious symbolism indicates the whole man and it is this that must unite in thinking, feeling and the will with the divine forces. Only the Christianization of the whole man can give the highest strength and it is this Christianization that brings the sword.

It is well known that the human organism needs iron. It is active in the red blood corpuscles and without it the human being would lose his power of resistance, become pale, passive and negative. Iron stimulates his activity expressing itself as warlike courage, but also in wild and quarrelsome behaviour. Spiritualizing the iron forces in the blood can however awaken spiritual initiatives. The presence of this spiritual, cosmic iron expresses itself in the growing human being as an indomitable will to inner freedom instead of a torpid resignation to convention and fate, and in a strong striving after knowledge rather than blind acceptance of what is taught. Mankind has lost the capacity to see how divinely beautiful this unbroken spirit-force can be in youth's unfolding. We must learn to look at it as the fairy-tale sees it.

The fairy-tale of "Iron Hans" points to this mystery. Near his palace a king has a mysterious wood. Many hunters disappear in it without trace until a brave hunter finds in the wood a pool, and in it a wild man with rusty brown skin and long hanging hair. The wild man, Iron Hans, is captured and locked in an iron cage in the palace courtyard. The king's eight-year-old son is playing with his golden ball and it slips into the cage. He asks Iron Hans to give it back and the wild man agrees if the boy will open the cage. The wild man even knows the place where the queen keeps the key, and finally the boy agrees to help. Freed, he takes the boy with him into the wood. There the king's son has to guard a golden well; nothing must fall into it and pollute its purity. Inadvertantly the boy dips his finger into the spring; then a hair falls in; finally his hair touches the water; and each in turn is changed to gold. The king's son has to go out into the world and experience poverty but his heart is pure and he is allowed one favour: in his greatest need he is to go to the edge of the wood and call "Iron Hans!" Then help will come to him: "My power is great, greater than you think, and I have vast stores of silver and gold."

Something fundamental is indicated here. In fairy-tales and sagas, boys — mostly when they are fourteen years old — are often called upon for wonderful ordeals and deeds. Perceval is the archetype of these "pure fools". He too is free of all connection with the world; his mother brings him up away from Church traditions and knightly customs in the isolation of the woods. When he is fourteen she lets him go out hunting alone but warns him to be careful if he sees anyone fully clad in iron. He is to cross himself against such people and run away. But when he sees five knights in full armour he believes they are angels of God and kneels in worship. This depicts the awakening of idealistic forces in the young human being. The image of the knight can awaken in a fourteen-year-old boy a presentiment of the divine mission which the human being has to undertake on earth. Nothing can hold him back; he tears himself away from his mother. She lets him go, dressed in fool's garb, and armed only with a javelin. And so he comes to a castle near the sea and under the castle gate sees a knight in red armour mockingly calling him to combat. Perceval, trusting to his innocent strength, fells the knight with his simple javelin, takes his armour and becomes the "red knight".

However ill-trained and foolish the pure-fool power may be on entering the human world, it is nevertheless given to it to succeed where many a battle-tried knight fails. The child can master the power that holds sway in the red blood-fire. As victor over the fire-forces, Perceval now succeeds in further adventures. Only because he has laid the red knight low can he free Blanchefleur (the white lily) in Belrapeire; and only because he has found her can he reach the castle of the Grail. For the Holy Grail is received in purified blood.

There are things that can go on in the soul which do not need to come to full consciousness in a young person. In the youthful soul they herald themselves in a storm of feelings and a presentiment of high human goals. The Grail vanishes from the soul again, to be sure; but the soul can seek the Grail anew in the struggles of its destiny and can find it again by knowledge painfully gained.

The boy in "Iron Hans" is only eight years old. At this age the iron in the blood appears at first in a different way. Around the time of the change of teeth, thinking frees itself and becomes eager to learn. A questioning that will not let itself be hemmed in by limits of knowledge, an insatiable urge towards the world in all its manifestations and the adventures it promises to the brave — all this often expresses itself with a certain impetuosity. For all iron radiation within human nature makes for activity but also for unruliness. This is uncomfortable for a world that does not like its well-ordered routine upset or its authority unsettled by questioning to which, for all its cleverness, it has no answer. For the king who has to guard his ancient heritage the "wild man" is a bit unsettling. He cannot just be killed; but by shutting him up in a cage the unsettling influence can be contained. The well-tried rules of upbringing, especially in an age of intellectual schooling, are nearly all designed to put "Iron Hans" under lock and key. It is inevitable that the boy should lose the golden ball to the man in prison; that the soul should find the fair gold of its childhood's dreams locked away. The key to opening the wild man's cage lies with the young soul-forces. Only a few will find these forces which do not surrender to the dictates of convention, lose courage to face unknown and untried paths, or renounce the urge to question the nature of all things. And where the world of rigid thinking gives no answer, the soul's own depths will.

The fairy-tale well in the depths if the will has not refused its gold. Mysteriously the glow shines and fascinates. But the soul that always looks only into its own depths falls in love with its own reflection like Narcissus. Then the well and the wood of dreams vanish. The fairy-tale gold cannot stand a greed that reaches for it or self-love that would only enjoy itself in everything.

The boy who had the golden well to guard but has sullied it is cast out into the world. He must now do Cinderella service. Even so, no-one can take from him his golden hair; it remains as a holy relic of his childhood's dream. But from now on he hides it with a hat.

The king's son begins his wanderings on beaten and unbeaten paths. He comes to the court of the king and works in the kitchen. The king rebukes him for wearing his hat while serving at the royal table and he is consigned to work in the garden. The princess catches sight of his hair and orders him to bring her flowers. It is characteristic that he chooses wild flowers instead of cultivated ones. "Wild ones have a stronger scent," he tells the gardener when the latter reproaches him. The king's daughter takes his hat off when he enters her room, looks at his golden locks and gives him a handful of ducats. He heedlessly gives the ducats to the gardener's children to play with.

The attitude of the soul to "gold" — both earthly gold and the gold of wisdom — is decisive for a wanderer seeking the spirit-light. The sight or thought of either kind awakens desire in the soul. Only by silencing the desire can the person rightly receive the grace of the spirit worlds. Hidden sources of strength are opened to him. He learns to use forces which come only to souls that are purified from selfishness. He becomes a Magus of the Good.

The true Rosicrucians of the later Middle Ages — not those false alchemists who boasted of their gold-making arts — made it a fundamental rule never to apply the wisdom they had attained to the service of their personal vanity or comfort. The hiding of the golden hair, the renunciation of royal lineage by menial service, and the refusal to accept unearned gold — by which he retains his freedom with regard to his fellow men — are the marks of a true disciple of the Rose-Cross. The fitness to receive the highest cosmic forces, the shining of Michaelic will-powers into the human soul is bound to these strict conditions.

It was always a question of finding a starting point for spiritual endeavour. One had to learn to go back to the years of childhood when the soul's powers untouched by desire still held sway. The child within had to be discovered. If one wished to start with the heart's powers that could lead to victory over the blood, then one had to go back to about the fourteenth or fifteenth year, when feelings for the wide world first awaken. But if one wished to take as a starting-point the youthful powers of thinking that had not been dulled by school knowledge or led astray by egotistic calculation, then it was necessary to reawaken the childish thinking and naive feeling that can still be present in an eight-year-old.

This youth or boy in man remains cocooned in the soul's depths: one must call him to new life. He can emerge from the hidden formative forces of man's being and be reflected in an imagination. Then the Grail-imaginations of the "pure-fool" arise, or the fairy-tale pictures of the boy who freed Iron Hans, sat at the well, and was cast out into the world. After this comes the stages of purification indicated by the boy's menial tasks. Then the awakening to the spirit-deed takes place, and lastly the stages of the bestowal of grace from the spirit are depicted.

The fairy-tale narrates how the land is ravaged by

153

war. The king's army is in extreme difficulties when a knight with an ironclad squadron charges into the enemy ranks and puts them to flight. No-one in the king's army recognizes the knight and he disappears after the battle. But he is the gardener's boy who has called on Iron Hans for help. The battle won, the boy gives the troops back to Iron Hans and returns to his gardening job.

The king in man is in greatest need; the spiritual heritage of mankind is threatened. The earthly powers are stronger and would destroy it if a young, hitherto unknown spirit power had not grown up, a power which alone can help. The will, kept free from all desire, strengthened in its passage through the earth's depths, can call up the strongest world-forces. They are only waiting to serve the courageous in spirit.

These forces are slumbering in iron. Iron, however, holds sway in the red blood and permeates it first with the lower self-assertive urges. Only through a wisdom that is beyond all greed for gold can the inner iron be spiritualized to become a bearer of higher moral forces. It permeates man's being with spirit-courage. Rudolf Steiner has characterized this inner iron irradiation as a fall of shooting stars in the blood; this appears as the microcosmic counterpart of the great cosmic process of the meteoric showers that rain down to earth as iron. Man's freedom is founded in its depths upon the development of such forces. Real moral action would be impossible without this working of the iron in the blood.

The fairy-tale describes the threefold revelation of the vanquisher. The king orders a great feast to be held. The king's daughter is to offer golden apples as prizes; perhaps the unknown knight will then appear. The youth asks Iron Hans to grant him the apples. This is promised and Iron Hans gives him red armour and a chestnut horse. On the second day of the feast he appears in white armour riding a white horse and on the third day in black armour on a black horse. The king is not pleased that the winner of the apples never reveals himself, and has him pursued. In the chase he is wounded and his golden hair seen. The princess guesses his identity and confronts the gardener's boy who admits his role in the events and shows the three golden apples. Because he has saved the kingdom and shows that he is a prince, the king allows him to wed the princess. During the wedding banquet the doors open and a stately king with a great retinue enters. It is Iron Hans, freed from his spell. He embraces the youth and says: "All my treasures shall be yours."

The boy who once possessed the golden ball and lost it has now caught the golden apple. And so he gains the fruit of the Tree of Life that can make the being of man immortal. Here the true significance of the princess is revealed. She is the dispenser of the golden apples; she belongs to that kingdom from which mankind was banished after succumbing to the serpent. The princess is the eternal part of the human soul that has not been drawn into the Fall.

Only as victor may the youth reach out his hand to her. And he becomes victor because he was able to wait until the forces had become ripe in him. The victor over the fire-forces of his own blood reveals himself as the red knight. It is the Perceval stage that we find here again. Mastery over the pure thinking forces appears as a second stage in the figure of the white knight. Finally the descent of the spirit into the dark nature of matter, and with it the spiritualization of everything material, is the sign of complete victory: the black knight appears and must finally show himself. The spiritually awakened can be recognized unmistakably by the way in which they know how to master the earth from the spirit. Once he has purified his feeling nature as the red knight and has spiritualized his knowledge as the white knight, he can become the black knight only by completely Christianizing his earthly will. Only at this stage may he unite himself in marriage with the virgin. He celebrates the "royal wedding". At this wedding the leading spirit, whose true form has hitherto been hidden from him, appears in his all-embracing kingliness. The mediator of the cosmic will-forces that call to freedom reveals himself as the Lord of Iron: the Archangel Michael.

14

The mystical wedding

A significant trait in many fairy-tales is that when something impossible becomes possible, other doors open. The enchantment is dissolved when a person comes to love what is enchanted. "Perhaps a similar transformation might occur if man could come to love the evil in the world," Novalis adds.

Here we touch on the mystery of the "mystical wedding" of the Middle Ages. The wedding which St Francis celebrated with his cherished "Lady Poverty" is an example of this soul-endeavour which is reflected in significant fairy-tale pictures. There is "King Thrushbeard", who escorts the proud maiden out of her kingdom when her father banishes her, and as a beggar lives with her in poverty. He leads her through trials aimed at breaking her pride, until she is stripped of all her royal dignity and deeply humiliated. Then King Thrushbeard reveals himself and raises her to his rank. They celebrate the wedding while she appears in the most splendid garments for only through humbleness can the true beauty of the human soul really shine forth.

Even more graphically the fairy-tales "Thousandfurs" and "Cinderella" (or Ashputtle) depict the development of the glory which can follow menial service. These are stages of illumination which lead the human being out of the transient to a union with the eternal.

The motif of Thousandfurs' journey of suffering is quite different from that in King Thrushbeard. In both cases the princess refuses offers of marriage, in King Thrushbeard out of pride: the kings and princes are not good enough for her and she mocks them all. The virgin human soul objects to uniting with the exalted powers of the cosmos that would permeate and illuminate her. She is conscious of her separate existence. Lucifer, the spirit that would lead us to our own selfish light and our own selfish will, works in the soul. Her tragedy is the Fall of man from which she will only slowly be raised again.

For Thousandfurs, renouncing royalty and entering into earthly poverty is an image of sacrificing the ancient powers of wisdom. The story tells that her father the king has lost his wife with the golden hair and cannot find a second wife, so he decides to marry his daughter. She refuses and runs away.

The soul's ancient, original powers of wisdom have died away. The future powers which are growing up bear just as much light-power, but they have first to go through the earthly world to develop complete independence. They have to leave the realm of supersensory life, for it would be an infraction against the divine plan of evolution and therefore a sin against the spirit, if this young soul-power, destined to wakeful cognition, were to fall back into the old clairvoyant consciousness and make use of old spiritual forces. The young soul-power would become mediumistic, like Rapunzel. Therefore — and this was known by all the initiates who served humanity's advance — the soul's development had to be severed for a time from supersensory experience. The soul-power had to take all spiritual-cosmic forces into itself and wait until they could unfold in a new way out of the power of the newly freed self. At this stage the human being no longer knows his cosmic origin and experiences himself in a dying physical body.

In "Thousandfurs" the princess with the golden hair thinks of a ruse in order to escape from her father's kingdom. She asks him for a fur coat made of skins of all the kinds of animals in the kingdom. After blackening her face and hands with soot, she escapes in the coat at night. Tired, she creeps into a hollow tree. The king who owns the wood finds her asleep in the trunk of the tree. He and his huntsmen initially take her for a rare animal. She cannot remember her origin or name, so they call her Thousandfurs after her animal coat and take her with them to work in the kitchen.

The maiden in the hollow tree is a motif we find also in "Mary's Child". There it appears as an experience of earth-maturity. The girl is fourteen years old when she is cast out of heaven. This is the age when earth-consciousness awakens fully within the physical: in the "hollow tree". The Tree of Knowledge is a picture of the nervous system, which branches out downwards from above. The system has become set and is dominated by death-forces: it is the hollow tree. In it the higher consciousness sleeps but the earthly consciousness is awake and feels itself permeated by animal urges. The senses can describe only a deceptive form of the human being. Only by overcoming this false picture can we become aware of the innermost: the spirit-personality, rooted in a moral existence. Gradually, with each cognitive advance, it can free itself and then a person finds his own archetype, woven out of cosmic forces, cradled in his true self. And if he tries to develop it then the supersensory form of man, in its connections with all the forces of the cosmos, begins to appear before him. A person can feel that the soul-life is still impaired by earthly urges and darkened by bodily needs, but if it can be spiritualized more and more, then the new and purer worlds of feeling will light up. This leads to the discovery of the purified "astral body".

Going even deeper into the being of man one can discover the life of the hidden formative forces that are active in all growth processes and in a refined state work in the forming of thoughts. These formative forces which, like all growth, are subject to certain effects of the moon, together constitute the "etheric body".

By penetrating to the very depths of the being of man one comes to recognize that the physical body cannot be a result merely of hereditary forces, but is built up out of the whole cosmos. Right into its individual organs and energy systems it is a microcosm, a reflection of all the stellar workings of the zodiac.

In every true cognitive endeavour ideas count for much less than deeds of awakening within the soul. The awakening takes place in three stages, revealing the mystery of the three sheaths which the human spirit has received from the cosmos, and at first bears unconsciously.

The fairy-tale indicates the same truths in pictures. It tells how the king's daughter asks her father for three dresses: one as golden as the sun, one as silver as the moon, and one as shining as the stars. Only when Thousandfurs finds that the king she serves as kitchen-maid is celebrating a great feast, does she appear in the dresses which she has kept hidden in a nutshell. Three feasts are held and each time she wears one of the dresses and dances with the king. Afterwards she puts on her cloak and blackens herself with soot. Then she serves the king a bowl of soup. The first time she puts a golden ring into the soup, the second time a little golden spinning wheel and the third time a golden bobbin: three precious things she had brought with her from her father's kingdom.

The soul which has led the sentient "astral body" to its purification — the dress as golden as the sun — can pledge herself to the spirit: she dedicates the ring to the king. The soul that has learnt to control the formative forces — the dress as silver as the moon — can think divine thoughts in unison with the spirit: she dedicates the golden spinning wheel to the king. The soul that has probed the mystery of the cosmic form of the physical body — the dress as shining as the stars — can extend her thoughts to the supersensory memory and so remember her origin in the divine cosmos: she dedicates to the king the golden bobbin on which single threads can be joined in long strands. When the king questions her about these events she denies all knowledge and says humbly: "I am good for nothing but having boots thrown at my head."

It was always known that the awakening of supersensory consciousness threatens at first to enhance the powers of pride and illusion in the soul. Thus we can recognize the true spiritual disciple by his readiness to immerse himself modestly each time in his earthly consciousness and practice humility with regard to his own self-esteem. Only the third stage of awakening leads to full cognition in the spirit; this is fulfilled in the royal wedding.

The fairy-tale of "Cinderella" chooses a different starting-point. It begins at the mother's grave. In the depths of the soul the primal wisdom lies sunk. At one time the human being lived in its light: from it he drew new strength, through it he was "rich". Since the time when the ancient wisdom was carried to the grave, winter has come to mankind. A covering of snow falls on the mother's grave. The world grows cold.

The fairy-tale tells how a rich man's wife lies dying and calls her little daughter to her bed. "Be good and say your prayers," she tells her, "I shall look down on you from heaven and always be with you." All through the winter the girl weeps at her mother's grave and remains good and pious. In the spring her father remarries.

Religion is but faithfulness to the "mother's grave": remembrance of the sunken wisdom in a time when the depths of the soul are covered with world-cold and darkness of intellect; faith in the all-presence of the soul of the world while the human soul is forced into service in the dust of the transient.

Cinderella must suffer the contempt of the proud stepdaughters. When the father asks them what he should bring them from the fair they reveal their natures, "Beautiful dresses," one of them asks for, "diamonds and pearls," the other, but Cinderella says, "break off the first branch that brushes against your hat on your way home."

In fairy-tales the aberrant powers of the soul are often presented as twofold. This reveals an intuitive knowledge that the human being can go astray in two directions: the Luciferic where pride and vanity work in the soul, and the Ahrimanic which leads to an inner rigidity where the soul is delivered over to the forces of matter. Between the two powers the true life of the soul is threatened with suffocation, unless it can enter into the depths of its being and there awaken higher powers. The mystic would say: There is still an innocent soul-power that has not been taken hold of by the Fall. This you must seek! It has appeared on earth through Jesus Christ, the new Adam. This is the branch that is sprung from the "Root of Jesse". It can

162

be planted in every human soul and there take root to grow into a tree.

In the legend of the "Hazel Branch" in the Grimms' collection, we are told how the Mother of God goes to look for strawberries in the wood for the Christ child. As she bends down to the finest strawberries, a viper springs out of the grass. The Mother of God takes fright and flees to a hazel tree and hides behind it. The viper creeps away. Since then hazel branches have been the surest protection against vipers, snakes and all other creatures that crawl on the ground. The snake lurks round the red berries growing on the ground, just as it lurks in the red blood. The hazel tree, on the other hand, stands for the truest life-force that could not be laid hold of by the Fall.

It is such a hazel branch that the father brings home from his journey for Cinderella, who plants it on her mother's grave. She waters it with her tears and it grows into a fine tree. Three times a day Cinderella sits under it and weeps and prays. And when she makes a wish, a little white bird perches in the tree and throws down whatever she wished for.

Christ says: "The heavenly Father [will] give the Holy Spirit to those who ask him!" In the Baptism in the Jordan the dove of the spirit alighted on Jesus, the pure offspring of mankind. Something similar is experienced by the mystic: the spirit's grace comes down to the soul when, in deep and regular meditation, the soul tends the power which is not darkened by any serpent, and whose roots can draw nourishment from hidden depths. From under the heart grows the purest offspring of life: the womb of the soul can become mother to this young power of God. The Christian mystic would say that in our hidden depths of soul "Mary" dwells.

Again the king, as in "Thousandfurs", holds a three-day feast so his son can choose a bride from the maidens of the land. All are invited. But the decisive question in this fairy-tale is whether the daughters have dresses fit for the wedding. The arrogant step-sisters make themselves as beautiful as they possibly can, but Cinderella is not allowed to go with them because she has no dress or shoes. She continues to ask permission and finally her stepmother agrees, but she sets a condition: she scatters a dishful of lentils in the ashes and gives her two hours in which to pick them all out. A will to do the impossible is a characteristic of fairy-tale heroes and the most touching virtue of their heroines. The girl calls out: "O tame little doves, O turtledoves, and all the birds under heaven, come and help me put the good ones into the pot, the bad ones in your crop."

It is a matter of being able to distinguish: a test of the power of judgment. It was always regarded as a fundamental condition of inner soul development that the disciple of the spirit should learn to distinguish strictly between the essential and the non-essential: to sort out the eternal from the transient. Our fairy-tale describes most beautifully how the white doves hasten to help. And then how, after the test has been successfully passed, the task is made more difficult but again accomplished. Cinderella is served by good powers. She has achieved "presence of spirit" in a literal sense. Even so the stepmother and her proud daughters will not take Cinderella to the feast, so she goes to the hazel tree and calls: "Shake your branches little tree, throw gold and silver over me." The white bird throws her a dress and shoes, she goes to the wedding, dances with the king's son who finds her most beautiful, but slips away back to her poverty before he can discover her name or where she lives.

The purification of man's being is revealed to

supersensory perception in the shining of the soul's garments. Every night when the soul-spiritual part of the human being rises out of the sleeping body, the soul's sheath — the astral body — begins to shine according to its state of inner development and spiritualization. The supersensory world then lights up for the spirit's gaze. The soul experiences a meeting with the higher self. The spirit-self seeks to unite itself with the soul.

The soul may have had a long contact with the spirit in the kingdom of the night without being conscious of it. These contacts can make themselves felt in moods and new resolves in everyday life. But the soul's power is not yet sufficient to carry over consciously what has been experienced in sleep. Generally the human being wakes up only in his head: sense-perceptions and concepts overwhelm the delicate impressions of the kingdom of the night, and the connection with the higher self is broken. There is however a higher awakening in the life of feeling; the nocturnal imaginations are supported by the finer nerve-system in which our subconscious dream-life takes place. But this too does not suffice to bring the spirit-world into everyday consciousness. Only an awakening in the depths of the will, which can grasp what has been experienced supersensibly, can enable the higher self to unite completely with the life of the soul. Now the soul must become aware of the golden trail of the supersensory when it awakens and hastens down the dark steps to re-enter the physical body. It must learn to bring to its perception what it has experienced and to do this at the very moment when that threatens to slip away.

The fairy-tale tells how Cinderella slips away from the king's son after he has danced with her: the first time through the dovecote which is an image of the head with unbridled thoughts flying about like doves; the second time through the pear-tree (the pear-tree and the apple-tree have been dealt with in connection with the "Girl Without Hands"); and finally she loses a golden shoe as she runs off down the staircase. Now the king's son seeks the maiden whose foot fits the shoe. The two proud stepsisters try to fit into the shoe, but their feet are too large. On their mother's advice they cut pieces off their feet, one a toe, the other a piece of heel. Though this device deceives the king's son, the doves in the hazel tree by the mother's grave tell him "there's blood in the shoe," and he realizes his mistake. Eventually Cinderella, who has been kept hidden from the king's son, tries the shoe. It fits, and he recognizes his true bride. The doves in the hazel tree confirm it when he rides past them.

There is a deep meaning in this testing of the foot by the king's son. How a man places his foot on the ground and how he walks shows his connection to the earth. It is significant whether he treads more with the toes or more with the heel when he walks. There is a tread which pushes the earth away too much and another which clings to it too much. Here again we see the twofold aberration of the soul which threatens man's being. Only a tread which has overcome the earth and can move over it evenly and rhythmically is the tread of the liberated soul. It becomes the dancer because it has vanquished the "spirit of heaviness". A human being's true maturity, his connection with the supersensory worlds — a connection borne by the spirit of Christ — can be unmistakably recognized by his relationship to the earth.

When the king's son rides away with his bride, the two doves settle on her shoulders. Thus the fairy-tale reaches its peak, like the "Tale of the Three Languages" in a Whitsun mystery. The soul which is beginning to unite with the higher self is raised to the level of inspiration. In the sense of Christian mysticism one could speak of the indwelling of the Holy Spirit in the inmost part of the soul.

The two sisters who with "blood in the shoe" tried to gain the prince's hand by fraud are condemned. On the wedding day the doves peck out their eyes. The soul that enters the spiritual world is blind if it has not yet overcome the lower sensual nature, and while not purified tries to force its way into union with supersensory life. It falls into even greater darkness. The fairy-tale teaches no fond illusions of the way to the spirit; it rejects all egotistic desire for the supersensory world. To grace it adds, most fittingly, the deepest earnestness.

15

The Virgin Sophia

"Cinderella" and "Thousandfurs" show the trials of
the human soul endeavouring to make itself worthy to
receive the spirit. In other fairy-tales it is more the
self, the human spirit striving and thirsting for self-
knowledge, that seeks to win back the pure archetype
of the soul. In the first case a starting point which
concerns the feeling is indicated, and from there the
soul can enter on the path of mystical deepening. In
the second case the stories point to a riddle of
knowledge which stimulates the thinker to investigate
the world and explore the formation of his own inner
being. Such a path of initiation appears before us in
pictures of solemn beauty in the fairy-tale of "Faithful
John". It leads us straight to the guardian figure who
holds the key to infinite mysteries. He is the hidden
teacher and inspirer of our fairy-tale world who shows
the young king his heritage, leading him to his palace
so that the king may become conscious of his glorious
treasures. This teacher is called John.

While the ecclesiastical tradition of the Middle Ages
speaks of "Peter holding the keys", the wisdom that
speaks in the fairy-tale pictures tells of "John holding
the keys". This wisdom is a witness to esoteric Christianity, for while Peter received the commandment
from the risen Lord to "feed my sheep" — to found the
Church — the other disciple, whom the Lord loved, is
given a different bequest. He hears the words from the
Cross: "Behold thy mother!" The Gospel adds: "And

from that hour the disciple took her to his own home."
These few words indicate an intimate experience in
the soul. Even in later Christian times many hearts still
endeavoured to follow inwardly, in deepest meditation, the stages of the Passion until they could stand
beneath the Cross, where they experienced "the
mystical death". As the lower nature was dying, the
soul opened to receive a higher mystery. The mystic
became himself a John and was able to take the
"mother" to himself, but he called her the "Virgin
Sophia". In his lectures on the Gospel of St John,
Rudolf Steiner points out that the Mother of the Lord
is never mentioned by name, but under the Cross she is
entrusted to one disciple as the most holy bequest.
Never, however, does John call her Mary. What John
honours by his deepest silence is expressed in images
in other early Christian writings. They speak of the
"Mother in the Heights", Sophia, who was also the
dove. In their writings the Risen One says to the
earthly Mary: "My mother in matter — thou in whom I
dwell." The Christian Gnostics tell of the fate of the
Light Virgin, of her descent from heavenly heights,
her wanderings in the world of matter, her call to the
divine spouse and her home-coming through Christ.*

The remains of that mystical literature, suppressed
by the Church, gives us some idea what the Light-
Virgin Sophia meant in the first Christian centuries.
Thus the great myth of her path of sorrow comes to us
in the ancient writing *Pistis-Sophia.* This myth is here
woven by the Risen One himself into his teaching of
the kingdom of light which he gives to his disciples. As
the virgin sought the veiled treasure of light, the
robber of light made it appear that what she sought
could be found only in the depths: her gaze was

* The Eleusinian mystery of the rape of Persephone and her rescue by
Dionysus has passed into transformed Christian mysticism.

directed downwards and, deceived, she made her way down into the world of desire where her own light-being was completely darkened. But Christ heard her call and came down. With his own path of sorrows he set before mankind, step by step, the mystery of purification. What had been sought since ancient times in the mystery centres — the great "catharsis", the purification of the soul — by single individuals, could now be found by everyone in following the stages of Passion. Pain, endured in freedom, transforms the soul into radiant wisdom. Once more the gates of the upper worlds, behind which the golden treasures of life lie veiled, open themselves to the soul irradiated with wisdom. It is this soul that attains the "treasure of light", which has the power to recreate all existence, and reveals to its possessor the mystery of the resurrection. "Wherefore, says the Risen One, you shall preach to all the race of man and say: Cease not, neither by day nor by night, to seek after the mysteries that purify until you have found them." Whoever finds them, receives also the pure Virgin Sophia.

In the wisdom of the Manichaeans of the third and fourth centuries this light-mystery lived on. Although the Manichaeans were publicly suppressed and proscribed, they maintained their secret knowledge in hidden ways and it flowed into the fairy-tale pictures. From them we have the princess of the golden castle, who is won by the prince in the tale of the "Golden Bird", and the princess from the castle of the golden sun, whom the youth with the "Crystal Ball" has to free.

The human being's memory of his cosmic origin in light is revealed in these virginal figures. In these pictures is reflected the knowledge that only one part of our human nature has been able to enter into incarnation: the other part — our "better half" as it were — has had to be left behind in the sunlit heights. This half is the "eternal feminine" that belonged to us from the very beginning, but which, because we have become entangled in earth-desire, we have forgotten. That is the cosmic adultery which earth-humanity has committed. The awakening of supersensory spirit-consciousness is a rediscovery of one's self in one's true being. All earthly union of man and woman in its noblest form can be only a transient symbol of it. It is then a life of repeated awakening from soul to soul, a life in which the souls bring to each other their archetypes. In all other cases earthly love can signify only an "enchantment" in which a sense-picture fills the soul-space where the archetype ought to appear. Then the power of passion sucks the idealistic feelings of the soul to itself and devours them.

In the "Crystal Ball" a difficult trial is laid before the youth who can see the king's daughter only with "human eyes", and so sees her as ugly and withered. He has to kill a wild bull which stands by a spring. Out of the bull rises a firebird which bears a glowing egg. Inside is hidden the crystal ball that can break the magic spell and allow the king's daughter to be recognized in her true beauty and glory.

The soul whose deepest fountain is darkened by lower passions cannot reach its supersensory archetype. In the quest for wisdom the soul finds at first only the sense-bound knowledge in which death-forces are working. Only when, out of waves of feelings and urges the soul manages to crystallize clear thinking can it discover a new life-centre within. Out of fiery burning egotism the chaste kernel of the self is released as a supersensory force-form. The soul gains the crystal ball. Through the purifying effect of the powers of thought the lower sense-knowledge is overcome and transformed back into radiant wisdom.

In the Persian Mithras mysteries, which the Roman legions spread throughout the Roman empire, the vanquishing of the bull by the hero is central to all ordeals of the spirit. This is a form of Michaelic deed which conforms with the ancient Persian wisdom. It is echoed in this fairy-tale picture.

In its clear-cut imaginations the fairy-tale of "Faithful John" (or Faithful Johannes) presents a knowledge of the laws of supersensory life. An old king who is dying sends for his best-loved servant, faithful John, to come to his bedside. He confides his anxiety about his son. Faithful John is to instruct and guide the lad. The king's son is to be taken to see his inheritance, all the rooms of the palace and the stored treasures: "But you mustn't show him the last room on the long corridor, where the portrait of the Princess of the Golden Roof is hidden. If he sees that portrait, he will be overcome with love for her. He will fall into a faint and later on he will face great perils for her sake; you must protect him from that."

Faithful John promises the king and undertakes his commission. Eventually the son demands that the locked door be opened and he sees the portrait. He resolves to win her for his bride, and faithful John has to devise ways and means of bringing them both into the presence of the princess.

With its descent from the spirit-heights mankind has lost that primal consciousness which could feel itself as king of all the treasures of creation. The ancient spiritual powers died away. But leaders and guardians of the divine heritage arose, and to them the keys of the mysteries of life were entrusted. By direct commission from the death-bed of the old king, from the spiritual powers that are dying out of earth existence, a

173

person is called to the service of mankind and is consecrated to his mission. A heavy responsibility is laid upon his soul. His service begins when he encounters another man's search for knowledge. He leads the disciple through the treasure-chambers of the ancient store of primal wisdom. He tells him that this is his heritage. The seeker after knowledge becomes conscious of his exalted origin and being observant becomes aware that the ultimate remains closed to him; not all the treasures are enough for him if he cannot see the picture in the locked chamber. A question concerning the mystery, coming from the depths, has power to make the guide open the door of the sanctuary. But from the truth seen in the picture, from an inkling of the truth, a force goes out that threatens to cripple all the life-forces when it strikes a soul which is not ready. The soul has prescience of a higher condition of life that is radiant in the gold of wisdom, and its beauty wakens in him forces of love previously unknown. This encounter with the ideal of wisdom kindles an enthusiasm with elemental violence that is the sign of the true discipleship. For him the guardian of the "Light-Virgin" can open the way further for that is his duty according to spiritual law.

True seekers of the spirit found in St John a guide to the mysteries when they meditated upon his words. He could stand before them as a living guide for the soul. United with his guiding power, the soul can find the way beyond the written word into the free kingdom of the spirit. The fairy-tale clothes the ordeals of the soul in the pictures of an adventurous voyage. In order to enter into the presence of the Princess of the Golden Roof the young king has one of the five casks of gold he has inherited from his father made into fantastic objects and loaded on to a ship. Then he and faithful John, disguised as merchants, set sail for the distant

city. The servant entices the princess on to the ship and
while she stands lost in wonder before the golden
works of art, the ship sets sail. Only when they are far
out to sea is she aware of the abduction and is at first
not to be comforted. But as soon as the young king
reveals his true lineage and his boundless love, she
gives her heart to him.

To reach your archetype protected in supersensory
regions, you must first create within yourself fitting
concepts which can give you the power to bring — one
might almost say capture — the content of the spiritual
world into your consciousness. Your archetype dwells
in the radiant element of wisdom. You must seek in the
soul's depths what is related to this element, and you
will find there a rich heritage of wisdom. Past cultures,
or to be more exact five great epochs, have worked to
fashion man. They have contributed their "five casks
of gold", working to infuse mankind with those spirit
forces which you can call up again. If you take hold of
these spirit-forces that belong to you, and in inner
activity use them to carve out a new realm of concepts
related by their inner nature to the spiritual world,
then your eternal self will give itself to you in the
beauty of its revelation.

But now the real ordeals of the soul begin. The
seeker after knowledge cannot avoid them. On the
voyage home, three ravens fly over the ship and tell of
the dangers that await the young king. When he lands
a chestnut horse will spring towards him; if he mounts
it will carry him off in the air. When he enters the
palace he will see a beautiful shirt shining like gold and
silver laid out before him; if he puts it on, it will burn
him down to the bone, for it is made of pitch and
brimstone. At the wedding dance his bride will turn
pale and sink down out of his arms. But each time he
can be rescued. A man who knows can shoot the horse,

throw the shirt into the fire, raise the bride and suck three drops of blood from her right breast and spit them out. But if he gives away his knowledge, he himself will be turned to stone.

Faithful John understands the language of the birds and determines to save his master. But his soul mourns for he feels disaster approaching. The prophecy is fulfilled when they land, but John is prepared for each trial. The other servants slander him and the young king, who cannot see why his guide has acted in this way, condemns him to the gallows. Before the sentence is carried out the faithful servant reveals the reasons for his actions and is turned to stone. In deep remorse the king has John set up beside his bed. Whenever he looks upon him his only wish is to bring him back to life. The queen bears him twins. One day while they are playing by his feet, John speaks: "You can bring me back to life, but you must sacrifice what you love most in the world." The king is ready to make the greatest sacrifice: he beheads his children and smears John with their blood. John is brought back to life and rewards the king's fidelity by resurrecting the children.

Ravens in myths and fairy-tales often bring messages from the earth to someone living in spirit-worlds. Faithful John, leading the young king from the other shore of existence back to the sense-world, listens to the laws governing spiritual experience when that experience is to be united with earth-consciousness: "Look, he's taking the Princess of the Golden Roof home with him. But he hasn't got her yet," say the ravens. That is a spirit-conversation behind the threshold of everyday consciousness, intimated to the initiate. He learns that everything experienced in supersensory realms is threatened as soon as it begins to mingle with bodily consciousness; it is extinguished, pervaded by illusions that distort pure spiritual vision. The "landing" brings dangers.

The human spirit can rise into realms of spiritual experience but the urges of the blood tend to take hold of it in day consciousness and cloud its vision: like a horse, they can run away with the rider. Wishes and desires introduce compulsive thought forms when the supersensory mingles with passionate elements in the soul. Waking cognition must maintain firm control over the blood in such moments.

When the spirit-seeker is freed from his body and looks down on it, he sees the formative life-forces glistening with the wisdom that was once active in forming his body. He feels deeply drawn to this, and longs to slip into the shimmering "shirt". But he cannot see that these formative forces, through their union with man's sense-nature, are burdened with wishes and drives and darkened with matter: the pitch and brimstone in the fairy-tale. The delicate forms in the supersensory consciousness are burned up by contact with these forces: hallucinations thrust their way in unless the magical power of the false shining is overcome.

Even if the seeker succeeds in uniting spiritual experience with earth-consciousness to remember the spiritual worlds, he will inevitably meet a third setback. There will be a tendency to clothe the spiritual reality in flesh and blood images. He tries to imagine spiritual reality as tangibly as sense reality and so altogether fails to catch the higher element in which ideas really live. Faithful John must suck drops of blood from the bride who is turning pale; only then can she win through to the life that is free from urge and illusion.

The marriage with the divine life has now been attained. This life imparts itself at first to human consciousness in the form of pure thought, but to the seeker this pure world of ideas does not feel warm and full of strength, but cold and dull. He cannot forgive his spiritual guide who has destroyed the illusory concept of the supersensory which he had formed out of his wishes. Spiritual reality has been divested of the sense perceptible to give him the purest form of knowledge, but his faith in his guide is deeply shaken. Doubts gain power over his soul and he cuts himself free from his guide. Modern man's endeavours in philosophy and science can be seen, in a certain sense, as a path of initiation. It is a spiritual development which seeks to enter the realm of pure thinking and is masked by the attainment of conscious individuality. The spiritual powers which formerly led the human being to knowledge and freedom are now forced to justify themselves before independent man. Mystery-wisdom is handed over to the executioner. If it is to make itself understood in its true nature, it must descend completely into the forms which modern intellectual humanity inhabits. Earth-consciousness lives in the mineral world. Into this mineral-like consciousness the guardian of higher wisdom must also descend if he is to make his actions comprehensible and present his mysteries to human judgment for testing. He himself must "turn to stone".

The living revelation of the spirit cannot be imparted in the way it was in the past: it is petrified, as it were, into a statue. To be reawakened it requires a counter-sacrifice, a deed out of innermost freedom by the person who has rejected the old kind of guidance.

A young force is born out of the union of man's striving towards wisdom and the light-filled spirit reality which at first shines in the inmost part of the soul only as a world of ideas. This force is the new self that has its being in both cognition and action. This twofold force — the twins in the fairy-tale — emerges out of the deepest personal experience, but must overcome everything: in the fairy-tale image, blood must flow. What the seeker is ready to give up of himself profits the supersensory life. The guiding being, the revealer, is liberated from the petrification of death which lies like a magical spell over all abstract thinking. He turns into a living inspiration. John, as an eternal figure of the spirit, is released from the magic spell and stands before the consciousness of the transformed seeker once more as the inspirer. A relationship, founded on freedom and sacrifice, between the awakened human spirit and the wisdom-filled guidance of humanity can arise. Then the rebirth of the mysteries can come about. They bring in a "Johannine Age" where the cognitive powers will be resurrected through an enduring sacrifice of the heart to them.

With prophetic power the fairy-tale delineates the destiny of all human spiritual endeavour. It unveils the goal of the person who strives for cognition — the Virgin Sophia — and the guardian of the most holy bequest — John who kept faith with his master. The bridal journey to the Princess of the Golden Roof leads to the threshold of that age whose dawn was prophesied by Novalis:

> Past is the long dream of pain,
> Sophie is the eternal priestess of the heart.

16

Observations
on some motifs

1. Educational points of view

Fairy-tales have a profound influence on the developing mind of the child. They envelop the soul in a magic
which is a necessary and healing counterweight to the
increasingly powerful effects of a technological society
in which children become intellectual and awake to the
earth far too early. Bringing alive the many different
moods in the telling or artistic presentation of fairy-
tales stimulates the powers of listening and feeling in
the soul and this is one useful way of developing
concentration in children who flit from one impression to the next.

We reach a proper connection to the characters of
the fairy-tale only when children themselves demand
the same thing to be told over and over again, just as
very young children can never hear enough of the
"Wolf and the Seven Young Kids" or try to act the story
of "Little Red Riding Hood". These characters can
often become vivid companions like the doll which the
little girl looks after and protects with such motherli-
ness and care. Of course she knows that the doll is not
"really alive", but she endows it from the full power of
her imagination with everything that can heighten its
reality. Basically the children never doubt the inner

truth of what is offered nor the existence of the fairy-tale heroes and heroines, as long as the narrator is really united with the truth-content of the fairy-tale. But because many parents and teachers can no longer bring an intuitive experience of the truth in the stories they tell, children begin to adopt a sceptical attitude to fairy-tales much too early.

For the healthy development of the soul it is of the greatest importance to present to the child a vision of an ensouled nature in order to counteract the mechanistic world-picture into which children grow all too soon. We must help the child in these early years, for the more tender powers of the soul experience a shock on meeting the ghostly treadmill of a soulless world; they shy away from it. A feeling that the world is not soulless can be induced by introducing the children imaginatively to the life and activity of the nature spirits. We should be able to talk about their habits and activities when showing a child the garden or walking through the woods and meadows.

Objections are often made to folk-tales on moral grounds. In the preface to their complete edition, the Grimms address this question. They stress the inner purity that pervades these poetic compositions and would have the collection regarded as an "educational book": "We do not seek that purity which can be attained by a pusillanimous expurgation of all that may pertain to certain circumstances and conditions which appear in daily life and cannot be concealed. By attempting such a purity we should be victims of the illusion that actions and happenings which are possible in the printed book must also be possible in real life. We seek the purity that lies in the truth of a straightforward story which keeps nothing wrong concealed. At the same time we have carefully eliminated any expressions which are not suitable for children. If it should then be objected that the parents may still be embarrassed by this or that, or find something objectionable so that they should not wish to let the book come into the hands of the children, there could perhaps be some foundation for this in isolated instances in which case the parent may make a selection, but in general this is certainly unnecessary. Nothing can defend us better than nature herself, who has caused flowers and leaves to grow in certain forms and colours; anyone who does not find them compatible with his particular requirements cannot demand that they should be differently coloured and cut ... Moreover, if we place the Bible at the head of all those sound and sturdy books that have nurtured our civilization, we know of none of them where such reservations are not present in even greater degree; but the right use will find no evil in them."

It is felt that children learn too much cruelty through fairy-tales, especially in the way that the punishment of the wicked is depicted. Children, however, have a feeling for natural justice which allows them to approve the correctness of a judgment based on spiritual laws.

There is also a concern that descriptions of the dark powers fill the child's mind with fear. But generally the cause of this lies in the mood of those who are telling the fairy-tales. One should be able to present convincingly the triumph of the divine that makes use of the humble, faithful and pure in order to establish its sovereignty in the realm of earth. Moreover the narrator with the right feeling will be able to counterbalance the deep earnestness of the tales with descriptions of humorous situations. The question of cruelty is also one in which the attitude of the narrator is deeply concerned. The tales should be presented with the earnestness appropriate to the profound truths contained in them, and this attitude precludes any sensationalism in the descriptions of punishment. It is, however, still tempting perhaps to avoid the darker tales, to veil the dark and questionable side of reality from children. But to do this is to risk producing adults whose capacity to bear life's full reality is weakened and who are prone to illusion.

The picture presented in the fairy-tales of the "wicked stepmother" can also present difficulties for the story-teller. Such a picture could implant in the child's soul prejudices which might make the task of a second mother endlessly difficult. Here we must assert that the fairy-tale takes its pictures from life's realities. It is not easy, even with an honest effort, to replace a mother. Good intentions and a right attitude are not enough. When destiny sets such a task, it can be accomplished in a conscious relating to the invisible presence of the dead mother. If anyone wishing to take the place of a child's mother avoids talking to the child about the dead mother, she will always encounter difficulties in bringing the child up. People who have died, especially a father or mother, wish to be taken consciously into the relationships of earthly life. If people make themselves open to the dead, in thought and attitude, they will be able to experience their helping power. A "stepmother" in the fairy-tale sense is one who places herself to block out the true mother, so that the true mother can no longer influence our world. Indeed it is in this way that the whole material world spreads a veil of darkness between us and the divine world so that we forget our spiritual homeland. Materialism acts towards our eternal being like a "wicked stepmother". When one is able to cultivate the right connection with those who have died, one is also able to find the words that will create trust for children in such situations of destiny.

When the young soul has come to the age when rightly the question of whether fairy-tales are true is raised, because the need for causal explanations begins to make itself felt, the right words must be found to allay the doubts. But one should not provide an answer that analyses the deeper wisdom of a fairy-tale. Often it is enough to indicate that besides the world in which everything goes according to strict natural laws, there is also another realm in which the soul has its true home. One can tell about those favoured individuals for whom the gates to this wonderful kingdom were opened. Let it be supposed that in former times such individuals were to be found more readily, often in simple guise and living in lonely places, as indeed the fairy-tales themselves recount; that even today there are such people and that the world could not go forward without such wise men and women. It does the child's soul good to awaken its feelings of reverence by imparting the idea that the best kings are those who wear invisible crowns, and that it is a blessing when such people walk upon the earth even today. Perhaps it may even be given to us to meet them somewhere? And a blessing on us if we can recognize them at the right time, despite their unimposing earthly guise.

2. The mystery of the horse

In the "Goose Girl" the princess's steed Fallada is always referred to as a horse. The Grimms however gathered another version of the conversation between the princess and the horse's head: "O foal, there thou hangest, O lovely maiden, ..." This suggests that the linguistic origin of Fallada has some connection with foal. Roland's horse is called Valentich, and Faland (or Valand, Voland) was a name used for the devil. In folklore it is held that the devil can always be recognized, even when he appears in human form, by his horse-hooves.

In the Younger Edda it is told how Loki changed himself into a mare and gave birth to a foal that was to become the best of all horses: Sleipnir, Odin's horse. This is a power that works as instinct, holding sway in the blood. It is Luciferic in nature, but still guided by the spirit and of service to Odin. The horse, at one time revered in the northern myths, turns more and more into a picture of the lower cleverness: indeed, the devilish cunning that leads mankind astray.

Here we see (as in the horses of the Apocalypse) a picture of the evolution of the intelligence. At first it works in the human being as a wisdom-filled instinct. In ancient cultural epochs the soul could not manage thought in freedom and was guided and taught by a deep instinctive wisdom. Thus arose the imagination of the centaurs. The centaur Chiron was the wise teacher of the Greek heroes; it was not human reason which spoke out of him, but the wisdom rising out of nature-urges.

This stage, when the human being was still intertwined with the horse, had to be overcome. The human being had to become the rider, learning to guide the horse himself, and master the instinctive wisdom forces with the power of his own self. The attitude of mind that determined his thinking was revealed in the colour of his horse: white, red or black. In the fairy-tale of "Iron Hans" these stages are very clear. In "Faithful Ferdinand and Faithless Ferdinand" it is a talking white horse that gives the youth wise counsel. Similarities are found in the Swiss fairy-tales, in "Bearskin", and its variation "Count Goldhair" in which the white horse, held captive in the stable of the devil, is carried off by the youth in an audacious ride. The horse gives him wise counsel and finally leads him to victory.

In the Breton fairy-tale of "Peronnik" which appears as precursor to "Perceval", the hero has to obtain a young foal in order to overcome all dangers. This foal belongs to the magician Rogéar, who rides past every day on a black mare. An important point is that the foal has not been shod, and is "a foal without a bridle". This indicates a childlike, untrained soul-ability, untouched by any intellectual education. Peronnik himself echoes this theme, appearing as the "simpleton" who, because of his untutored nature, can still rely on the heart's assurance in all situations.

The southern Swiss story of the "Thirteenth Son", the "Tredeshin", has a horse "as white as fresh snow and as swift as the wind". This horse belongs to a magician, but is so much desired by the king, at whose court Tredeshin is serving that the king falls ill. Whoever can bring him the horse shall receive the princess as wife and half the kingdom as well. The snow-white steed is guarded by grooms in the magician's stable; also they guard the black steeds with blood-red nostrils. The grooms represent the human senses: they keep the dark passions tethered, but also guard the snow-white steed. Tredeshin can approach the magician's dwelling only in the evening and he steals the white horse by sending the grooms to sleep. This white steed indicates an ability which remains hidden within sense-existence during the waking hours. Without this ability, the spirit in us cannot feel itself to be truly a king, however great the kingdom he rules over. The language of the fairy-tale indicates a power of thought which can move about in the kingdom of the spirit free of the fetters of the senses. This power of thought must be transferred into the possession of the spirit. During waking life our thinking is at first bound to the body and our concepts move within the limits of the sense world. But if they can be freed at the moment of going to sleep, when sense-experiences begin to fade, then the pure light of thought can carry the spirit out of the body's life. Tredeshin makes himself the bearer of these newly awakening abilities.

In the "Golden Bird" there appears a golden horse that can run faster than the wind. When the soul has freed itself from the sense-nature, it can let itself be borne along by world-thoughts, freed of space and time. Here a sun-initiation is indicated. Thought-powers, coming from pure realms of the sun, are ready to give themselves to the spirit of man. Only through them can he find the union with his higher self which has its being in spiritual heights. The king's son can bring the beautiful princess of the golden castle home only on the golden horse.

In the fairy-tale of the "Miller's Drudge and the Cat" the old miller promises to give the mill to the journeymen who can bring home the best horse. The two older lads think themselves very clever, but one brings home a blind nag and the other a lame one. But stupid Hans, who has served the cat for seven years, returns with a splendid horse. A person may be very proud of his own view of the world, but faced with the riddles of existence this outlook can reveal itself as nothing but a blind or lame horse, unfit to carry its rider through life. When the intelligence is still acting instinctively, it can easily come to serve a lower egotism that becomes sophisticated and knows how to mask its aims while using every means available to achieve them. Nevertheless the "horse's hoof" is visible in everything he does. Psychoanalysis is fundamentally a science of the centaur, the horse-man who still lives deep in the human being. The instinctive wisdom of the subconscious life of the soul has become the creeping cunning of the desire-nature: the devil has a cloven hoof not a human foot.

3. Bearskin

The imagination of the bear appears where the human understanding moves in the heavy armour of the logical rules and "factual" proofs, or the strait-jacket of materialistic thought-forms. This human logic, which tries to dance yet cannot escape the heaviness of earth, appears absolutely ridiculous to the gnomes, who have an intuitive and total comprehension. Human thought, feeling its way along uncertainly, is for them a source of amusement.

For the seeker of the spirit, it may be necessary to go through the schooling of earthly thinking, with its exact methodology: he must slip into a bearskin. This image appears in the "Golden Children". A soul which has brought into earth life a wealth of shining gold must enter intellectual thought-forms for a while, if it is to maintain itself in a materialistic age. Similarly in "Bearskin" the soldier who makes a pact with the devil must wear a bearskin. If the human spirit devotes itself to natural science, it must make a compact with the Mephistophelean power. In order to learn how to master the forces of the earth, the human spirit must undergo such schooling, which at first entails a certain darkening and wasting of the soul-life — even though a person intends to use these forces of the earth for the good of humanity. Intuitive-artistic abilities will be stunted, and powers of the heart and mind will wither during this period. The fairy-tale says that the soldier (the fighter against evil) has to wear the bearskin, not wash, comb his hair, cut his nails or pray for seven years. The devil demands that the soldier leave his soul-life uncared for. Seen spiritually, a complete immersion in scientific endeavour and research, corresponding to the materialistic spirit of the times, results almost always in a devastation of the soul-life. It is always a risk for inner development. But the soldier may feel the spiritual risk to be worthwhile and he only needs to wear the bearskin for seven years.

In "Count Goldhair" the horse and the bear are placed next to each other. They both stand enchanted in the devil's stable. The youth who goes to "school" with him is to feed them, but when the horse begins to speak, he decides to free both animals. After they have escaped the horse commands the youth to kill the bear and wear the skin to hide his golden hair. The practice of humility is seemly for a shining soul striving towards wisdom. If a person intends to realize his ideals and spiritual abilities in accordance with modern demands, he must first patiently acquire the expertise of earthly reason and a knowledge of the science of the senses. The higher spiritual powers must for a time withdraw into the inmost intimacy of the soul. Thus the true disciple of wisdom appears to the world in a bearskin. Only when he has passed all the tests which will guarantee to the spirit a mastery over himself and the world of matter, can the bearskin be shed once and for all.

4. Trades in the fairy-tale

In the "Two Travelling Companions" a tailor and a shoemaker meet on the road. One is jolly and cheerful, the other with a face as if he had drunk vinegar, a fellow without a sense of humour. There is a heaviness in him. The tailor is usually depicted in fairy-tales as enterprising: in a good and bad sense he has a sanguine temperament. The shoemaker who makes firm soles for the earth underfoot is more ponderous, burdened as it were with the cares of the earthly path that man must tread. A real shoemaker knows how those whose shoes he mends tread on the earth. Their gait is revealed in the way they wear their shoes out. The human soul unites itself unconsciously with the earthly task; the shoemaker cannot help becoming melancholic or short-tempered. In the fairy-tale, the shoemaker appears as the dark double of the tailor; he portrays demonic forces seeking to infiltrate a light-filled soul so as to darken and pester it with evil suggestions.

Where the shoemaker, however, is filled with goodness of heart he will be able to take into himself the dark ways of other people's destinies and help them to become free. In Richard Wagner's *Meistersinger*, Hans Sachs, the shoemaker-poet is depicted as just such an initiate of the heart. He knows "just where the shoe pinches" each person. And because Jakob Böhme was a down-to-earth shoemaker, he did not get carried away, like many of the mystics of the Middle Ages. In deep thought he knows how to unite the light of Christ with the heaviness of the earth. He is constantly musing upon the riddle of evil, and why light should need darkness in order to manifest itself. We also meet such a shoemaker in the "Juniper Tree".

In the miller we meet someone who grinds away everything we receive as sense-impressions, transforming it into food for the hidden part of our being. We go through experiences and become wiser; we meet our fate and grow stronger. Anthroposophy speaks of the etheric body, which works within the physical, and like a hidden craftsman, fashions our form after the manner of the impressions and stimuli it receives from life. The Finnish epic, *Kalevala*, tells of the forging of a mysterious mill, the "Sampo", which symbolizes this etheric body. A higher consciousness, hidden within us, works in this etheric organism, and it can appear in the picture of the miller preparing food. But the soul that awakes in the kingdom of the etheric formative forces and learns to see the mysteries of the transformation of substances, experiences itself as the "beautiful miller's daughter" as in "Rumpelstiltskin".

In the "Miller's Drudge and the Cat" it is a question of who should inherit the mill. What stupid Hans has to learn represents a way of cognition. He achieves mastery over the etheric formative forces which build up the human being and are constantly transforming him. He is indeed working with silver tools on a silver house.

5. Fairy-tales of pixies

Some fairy-tales lead us into the kingdom of the water-beings: the undines and the nixies. They appear as beings who feel a longing for what is human. The beings of the elemental kingdoms long to be transformed and liberated by the pure powers of the human soul. The undines do not yet know what life in warm blood is and what can blossom from it. They are seeking to attain the power of love.

The fairy-tale pictures are illuminating in many ways. We sometimes find people who have an undine-nature. They live as if enchanted in the etheric world, innocent in feeling, but taking little part in the warmth of human living. Their inner life is inadequate. Often it requires some heartfelt experience before the spell is broken. The fairy-tales tell of the awakening of the powers of love and the transformation of the undine into a loving human, and this applies also to such hidden "nixiness" often found still in many human souls.

The marvellous tale of the "Nixie in the Pond" includes such features. A miller is tricked into promising his new-born son to a nixie. The boy grows up and experiences the great joy of deep love. But one day he is caught by the nixie in the millpond. The wife he has left behind is shown in a dream how to rescue him. She has to bring the golden comb, the golden flute and the golden spinning-wheel to the pond to obtain the release of her stolen husband.

Light of wisdom, offered by human love, effects liberation for the elemental worlds. The beings of the etheric world long for gifts of soul, gifts that are shining with spirit, offered from the human heart.

The fairy-tale mirrors processes of consciousness: enchantment and release. But it can also direct our vision to secrets of life after death. The loving wife sends spirit-help to the soul of her dead husband, for the soul needs such gifts of light while it is still under the magic spell of the undine. First the head, then the breast and finally the complete figure of the dead person emerge from the water. The awakening of the soul in the realm of the dead takes place in three stages.

Even so the loving ones are finally separated and have to undergo transformation before they again attain human form. They find themselves among strange people and sadness and yearning fill their souls. As luck would have it they meet again when a new springtime comes to the earth. They do not recognize each other but are glad that they are no longer alone. One evening, in the light of the full moon, the man plays a lovely sad tune on his flute and his wife recognizes him. Once she had played the tune by the millpond to free her loved one from the undine. Although they now have different forms, they recognize each other by the same melody.

Mysteries of transformation are revealed to the soul that can communicate with the water-beings. Goethe received his inspiration for "Song of the Spirits over the Waters" as he watched the Staubbach waterfall. There he learned the great mystery of the transformation of the human soul from one earth-life to another.

6. The mystery of winter

In the ancient Hibernian mysteries the neophytes were led to certain great landscape pictures. Rudolf Steiner describes how this imaginative experience leads first into a dying, solidifying world: winter landscapes with snow-flakes and ice-fields appeared to the neophytes as soon as he began to discover the nature of his sense-organs. On the other hand, the seeker saw summer pictures arise as wonderful dreams of nature when he no longer felt the complexity of his senses but felt himself as a unity, as though contained within the heart. And here the future was revealed to him. In the snow-crystals the powers of spirit, dying into matter, presented themselves to his imaginative vision, but in the summer dream-pictures the germinal forces of a future universe manifested themselves. The human being stood as mediator between a dying and a reborn world.

The fairy-tale of the "Juniper Tree" paints such a transition from a winter to a summer mood in an exceptionally poetical way. Against a similar background "Snow White" can be seen as a Christian experience of the passage of the seasons. From the falling snow-flakes the mood of Advent speaks to the soul as it waits for the divine child. It is ready to receive the immortal kernel. Then follows the transition to the Christian birth, and then to the mood of Lent and the Passion. From the deep-felt fateful mood of Good Friday it changes to the solemn calm of the burial, and in the awakening of Snow White from the glass coffin the soul's Easter festival is celebrated. In such an interpretation of the fairy-tale, the outer events are of less relevance than an inner calender of the soul which is reflected in the destiny of Snow White.

We find a significant exposition of the winter mystery in a fairy-tale on the theme of liberation, which resembles the "Lilting Leaping Lark" and the English fairy-tale of "Beauty and the Beast".

The story tells of a merchant asking his three daughters what he should bring them from the fair. One asks for a beautiful dress, the second for a pair of shoes, but the third asks for a rose, though this request seems impossible as it is winter. On his way home the merchant comes to a castle with a garden where it is half summer and half winter. He plucks a rose but as he is riding away a horrible black beast comes snorting after him and threatens his life. He manages to escape only by promising to give the beast his daughter, "the most beautiful girl in the world".

Even more profoundly this motif of the rose appears in the Swiss fairy-tale of the "Enchanted Prince". Here the father goes into an enchanted palace and finds the whole garden in spring blossom even though it is deep winter. He plucks the loveliest rose, near a fountain. For that he has to promise his youngest daughter to a ghastly serpent that appears out of the fountain.

In the language of Christian mysticism the blooming rose is a picture of the purified blood-nature of the human being. Thus it is always a mystic symbol of Christ's love. But in the fairy-tales it appears in a situation of deep contrasts: it blossoms in winter.

The miller who plucked the lovely rose for his youngest daughter had also to face the ghastly serpent which crept out of the fountain, where the glorious rose-bush stood in bloom. What the fairy-tale says is that whoever tries to understand the mystery of the rose must of necessity also encounter the serpent. The soul may not shun self-knowledge. First it must get to know the forces that still have power over the blood: the daughter must marry the serpent. Now the soul must find the courage to light a candle in the night and by the rays of higher knowledge release the being of the snake from its enchantment. These are ordeals of humility laid upon the miller's daughter which point unmistakably to the path of Christian mysticism whose highest goal is the transfiguration of the powers of love: the freeing of the serpent from its enchantment.

7. The apple

We can trace the motif of the apple through the myths and sagas of many peoples, as well as in its variations within the world of fairy-tales. The laws of the language of imagination can be demonstrated by the example of the apple. Well known are the apples of the Younger Edda, which Iduna keeps stored in a vessel; by eating them the gods can constantly renew their youth until the coming of the twilight of the gods.

These apples are the fruit of the Tree of Life denied to man after he had eaten from the Tree of Knowledge and so entered the sphere of death. There is a profound truth contained in the Nordic mythology that gives Bragi, the god of the skalds' arts, Iduna as wife. For it is poetry, the divine power of song, that constantly imbues mankind with the holy life-forces, and maintains a certain counterbalance to the intellectual development which is connected with the forces of ageing and death.

In Greek mythology, golden apples are guarded by the divine virgins in the Garden of the Hesperides, far away on the coast of the Western Ocean. Hercules, the hero striving for immortal life, has to undertake the journey to the Hesperides and bring back three apples. Here the saga points to a certain stage on the way of initiation. Atlas, the guardian of the Atlantean primal wisdom, undertakes the task for Hercules. This giant bears the dome of the sky on his shoulders, which means he still has that cosmic consciousness which bears the whole firmament as a memory within it. Clearly, Hercules has to acquire powers which mankind has lost in the course of evolution. These powers are guarded in far off consecrated places near sunken Atlantis. The golden apples signify the forces that renew life, forces which by divine decree must be kept from human desire, but must be obtained by the seeker who would awaken the immortal in himself.

The saga tells of a dragon that bars the entrance to the garden. The dragon must be put to sleep and killed before the tree can be reached. This Atlas can do, for the Atlantean still had the ability to go right back in memory to the pristine light. In grace-given moments the gates of paradise were opened to him. On the spiritual pilgrimage which leads Hercules to the gates of such a place of consecration, he must pass through ordeals of the soul. The vanquishing of the dragon signifies the victory over desire which masks the approach to the hidden mysteries of life. This saga is the archetype for a series of fairy-tales which in many variations describe the quest for the forces that rejuvenate life. A fairy-tale from Grisons (Graubünden), similar to the "Water of Life" tells of three golden apples which the prince has to bring to his sick father from the enchanted garden. A peasant comes to the court and tells of the enchanted garden and the golden apples. The peasant is a simple folk-figure, one of those people who have retained something of the old spirit knowledge. In this story the enchanted garden is entered at high noon, while in the "Water of Life" the mystery can be attained only in the stillness of night.

The soul is absorbed in worlds of light; in cosmic spaces the spiritual can be sought and found, but in a trial that takes place in the realm of night the way inwards into the depths of the human soul is indicated. So here the virgin by the fountain appears "as bright as the sun". It is the pure light-nature of man which the seeker after the spirit finds again in holy ether-realms. He has to release the virgin which means he must unite her with his own waking consciousness. But he is in danger of becoming captivated by the sweet songs of the birds in the garden, forgetting what he came for, and not noticing how time goes by. The seeker after the spirit must not lose himself in unworldly bliss or in the taste of paradisal joys. While he finds himself free of the body in the etheric world he must be able to keep awake the memory of earth and his human duties.

Similar motifs are found in the "Golden Legend" about Seth, Adam's son, who undertook a pilgrimage to paradise to obtain for his sick father healing oil from the Tree of Compassion, but was told by the Archangel Michael that the oil would be denied him for thousands of years until the Redeemer came to earth.

The image of the apple appears in connection with the awakening of the powers of desire at puberty. But it would be a mistake to regard this earth-maturity of the young person one-sidedly as sexual maturity. The young person at this stage becomes fully open to impressions from the sense-world for the first time. A new awareness of the opposite sex is only one manifestation of this comprehensive awakening of the soul that takes place on the threshold between childhood and adolescence, and is reflected over and over again in a wonderful way in the fairy-tale pictures. But one must recognize the heavenly origin of this surge of feeling, which can appear either fervently or wistfully. When the soul's full capacity for experience ripens it desires the fruit and is endangered by the powers of the blood that threaten to dominate. Then the soul's capacity for love becomes sensual desire which is out of keeping with its original nature. The sexual urge is in no way the true instigator of the capacity for love, but rather its perverter, for sexuality darkens the divine power of Eros and so the apple is "poisoned". The serpent has meddled with the experience of paradise.

When Snow-White is pursued by her wicked step-mother into the kingdom of the dwarves, and talked into eating the poisoned apple, she must die. "Snow-White longed for the lovely apple," says the fairy-tale, thus indicating the rousing of sense-desire. Snow-White is the chaste light nature that dwells hidden in the human being. Her body is incorruptible, as the dwarves know, and so they will not "lower her into the black earth". Though she may fall into a deep enchanted sleep, she will be reawakened out of her glass coffin to new life as soon as she is able to eject the poisoned apple that is foreign to her true nature. In this sense the apple can be taken as a picture of the selfish part of human nature. It symbolizes the self which has plunged too deeply into sensuality. It is no longer the "golden apple" which gives forth rejuvenating forces. This apple can be plucked only in hidden places by the person who has fought the dragon, or it can be given as a gift of grace to a youth like the gardener's boy in "Iron Hans", or, as in "Count Golden Hair", the youth who has proved that he has mastered the sensual.

By contrast, the fruit of the Tree of Knowledge is full of the workings of death. In gruesome fashion this picture of the death-bringing apple appears in the "Juniper Tree". It is told in a similar way in a Swiss fairy-tale "Little Brother and Little Sister". The mother sends her two children into the forest to gather wood. The child who comes home first with his burden is to get a beautiful red apple out of a chest. As he bends over, she lets the heavy lid fall and chops off his head. Again it is a process of development to which the fairy-tale points. The youthful urges in the soul, appearing as brother and sister, are on the way to becoming conscious. They are born from the senses. Accordingly the mother (nearly always called the stepmother) appears as the arouser of selfish desires. She invites the boy to reach for the apple, thereby killing the young spiritual will. She makes him head-less, that is, she casts him down into the shadowy birthplace of desires. The sister opens the trough in which her dead brother has been laid and a little white dove flies out. From resting in the death which the apples concealed, the dove of the spirit arises in liberated flight after the stages of suffering have been passed through.

8. The heavenly twins

A fairy-tale from Romania tells the story of two golden children born to a beautiful young woman. The jealous serving-maid kills them and lays a young dog in the cradle. The father casts out his wife and marries the maid. Two apple trees, with golden branches and golden apples, grow out of the hearts of the golden children. The maid has the trees cut down. But the father's sheep has eaten one of the golden apples and gives birth to two golden lambs. These the woman has killed but when her maid is cleaning the carcasses at the stream, the entrails are washed to the other bank and give birth to the two golden boys again. They grow quickly to radiant beauty. After finding their mother, they return to their father's house wrapped in beggars' clothing. He recognizes them and receives them with joy.

When the sunlike being of man, in its duality, is submerged in sense-existence it must experience death. But this being of man is indestructible: in the development of the human soul it only passes through transformations. The golden apple tree is indeed the Tree of Paradise, still shining with the primal light. But its fruits cannot be given in undiluted form to earthly man. They must first be led through sacrifice and experienced inwardly. The destructive will of the "maidservant" who has usurped the place of the bride of light tries to extinguish the sunlit wisdom, but she cannot destroy the wisdom completely. In a mysterious way the wisdom recreates itself as the lamb. This is an indication of the transformation of the original wisdom into the Christian mystery, through which it can be rescued and brought to rebirth.

Once the picture-world of the fairy-tales has revealed the twin nature of man's eternal being, an understanding of a great Christian mystery can come. In the Gospels of Matthew and Luke two quite different stories of the birth of Jesus are told. They remain a contradiction impossible to reconcile as long as we consider only one Jesus child. In his lectures on the Gospels Rudolf Steiner showed in detail that there were two children both called Jesus. One is born king of wisdom, to whose house the wise men of the East make their pilgrimage (according to Matthew); the other is the child of poverty, over whom the heavens open and at whose crib only the simple shepherds appear (according to Luke).

In the Matthew child we must see the incarnation of an individuality who went through his development at an earlier date and in whom all human culture is represented. The Luke infant is the eternal child who gazes into the world from the depths of a loving heart. As a unity, these two children present, for the first time, a complete human being. The Matthew child would be at the end of its development were it not rejuvenated at the hands of the other heavenly being.

Rudolf Steiner goes on to show how the two children seek and find each other and in a mysterious way become one human being, the bearer of the Christ-Spirit. Though it may sound strange and even repellent to religious feelings grounded in tradition, a new view of the being of Christ can grow out of a deeper and more comprehensive understanding of the laws of human development. Anyone who begins to understand the fairy-tale of the "Two Golden Children", or of the "Two Brothers" who go east and west, part, and in their greatest need hasten to help one another, will be able to approach the mystery of the childhood of Jesus in a new way. The mystical tradition has always been acquainted with it.

9. The ravens

Ravens play a significant part in Nordic folk-tales. From them the leading folk-spirit receives news of what is happening on earth. Odin sends out the ravens "Huginn and Muninn" (understanding and memory) into the world. Rudolf Steiner describes how the leading spirits send down a small part of their forces into the sphere of the senses when they need to work into the earthly world. When these forces are cut off and made independent, bird-forms arise. Zeus's eagle and Odin's ravens are the senses of a higher comprehensive spirit-consciousness, organs that extend into the supersensory life of the atmosphere. Through them a divine being investigates the periphery of the earth-world. Someone who has been snatched away by Zeus's eagle and borne up to the hall of the gods, as was Ganymede, has been taken into the life of the spiritual world. The transformation of the brothers into ravens means that part of the higher powers of wisdom is lost while individual consciousness develops. The ravens have their equivalent in the human soul, for the folk-spirit sends into it similar divine powers. So Odin endowed his folk with the power of thought and memory; a remembrance of the divine world which has sent us down into earth-existence as messengers. When the thought of life in spirit-existence dissolves and the memory of that exalted origin is torn away, Odin finds his ravens cannot find their way back to him. Therefore the wandering god in Grimnir's song in the Edda speaks the prophecy of doom: "I fear for Huginn that he will not return home, but heavier is my care for Muninn." The sacred original memory that was able to maintain the soul in community with the gods dies out; the twilight of the divine worlds sets in for the soul.

In the myth the god loses the ravens; but the fairy-tale has the human powers of wisdom transformed into ravens that fly away. These are two different views. In the myth the divine powers of thought and memory can no longer find their way home. For the gods it is a loss when human consciousness is estranged from the spiritual world. In the fairy-tale the emphasis is on the soul's development: the supersensory powers of thinking tear themselves away from the human being who is awakening to himself. They operate as "ravens" in the outer world, but no longer within the soul. The soul must learn to reawaken in itself the same forces that still weave and live on the earth's periphery. Then the soul will be able to ally itself anew with the divine guiding powers and will once again receive messages from the spirits.

In the "Twelve Brothers" it is the twelve cosmic senses that become ravens; whereas in the fairy-tale of the "Seven Ravens" a sevenfoldness of powers are described. This tale refers more to the soul-urges

203

which are born out of the "astral world". The girl finds her way into the world of the seven planets. The morning star — from ancient times the messenger of the gods and the star of spiritual illumination — gives her the key to the realm where she may rediscover her seven brothers, her supersensory powers of conscious-ness. Human thinking begins again to be permeated with the thinking of the gods.

Another Grimms story, the "Raven", tells of a little princess cast under a spell by her mother. Turned into a raven, the child hides in a dark wood. A man hears the raven's cry for help. She tells him that she is a king's daughter under a spell, but that he can release her. After various tests he finds her in a golden castle at the top of a glass mountain, impossible to climb. Even-tually he manages to climb the mountain and enter the castle invisibly. A significant feature in the story is how he sees the maiden sitting in the hall with a golden chalice filled with wine before her; he draws from his finger the ring which she had once given him, and drops it into the chalice. Recognizing the ring she knows that the man who will release her from the spell is close.

The human being's higher spirit-being has to lead a shadowy existence — to be turned into a raven and live in the enchanted forest — as long as the seeker after the spirit does not succeed in restoring his connection with it and awakening it to full life by moving it from the sphere of the head to that of the heart. This is indicated by the dropping of the ring into the golden chalice filled with wine. The connection with the ideal image is only a thought-experience to begin with and works on in the soul as memory, but for the liberation to take place it must be plunged into the heart's depths and from there, reborn. The mystery of the chalice is a sacramental picture of this.

10. The trinity of the soul's powers

Thousandfurs places the golden ring, the little spinning-wheel and the little bobbin into the king's soup,
linking herself secretly to him. We often meet in fairy-
tales three such magic gifts which express faculties of
the soul. To understand them in their imaginative
sense it is necessary to consider how each one operates.
The three gifts are always concerned with the trinity of
thinking, feeling and the will, or with spiritual mastery
of the three bodily sheaths in which the spiritual self
dwells. In the tale of the "Spindle, the Shuttle and the
Needle" these are the three magical implements that
are to bring the suitor to the house of the poorest girl
(who in fact is the richest). They represent the three
faculties of the soul which must be developed: thinking illumined by the spirit that must become active in
the soul (the girl is fifteen years old), for it to attain its
true self and learn to unite with the spirit; a wisdom-
filled feeling which can weave a dream of paradise
with an inner wealth of imagery; and an active will
purifying the whole of man's being, and able to
transform the body and soul into a dwelling for the
spirit. In the fairy-tale the spindle spins the golden
thread that follows the king's son and brings him to the
house; the shuttle weaves the costly carpet of pictures
over which the king's son may step as he enters the
house; the needle, aided by invisible spirits, decorates
the whole room with velvet and silk so that the suitor
may be fittingly received. Thinking, feeling and the
will are called upon to prepare the proper reception in
the soul for the mystery; then the "royal wedding" can
be celebrated.

Another trinity of talents is indicated in the fairy-
tale of the "Magic Table, the Gold Donkey and the
Cudgel in the Sack". A tailor's three sons leave home to

learn a trade, one a carpenter, one a miller, and one a turner. At the end of their apprenticeship each one receives a gift: a table on which food miraculously appears, a donkey that produces gold, and a cudgel which fights for its owner. The first two are atavistic abilities and anyone who reawakens them in the old way must be careful. They can become mingled with egotistic powers of the soul, resulting in illusions.

In other fairy-tales we have seen the magic cupboard of food which the golden fish gave to the fisherman and his wife. This, like the little table, is a very ancient talent which at one time was common to all mankind, but has grown dim with the development of our present consciousness. In our subconscious the cosmic is at work, taking into itself the nourishing forces of the universe with which it builds and regenerates the body. With an awakening selfishness in the human being this innocent, wisdom-filled part of our being had to be kept under guard; the whims of egotism cannot be allowed to gain access to the hidden life-forces and so interfere with their activity and spoil them.

The gold donkey represents a different instinctive capacity. Here we are dealing with ancient powers of wisdom completely bound to the physical and arising from inherited predispositions. The deeper we submerge ourselves in the earth-world, the more our traditional wisdom becomes adulterated by a darkening of foresight and confusion of dreams. The donkey spits gold; he speaks his wisdom out of his old inheritance. But a gift that is no longer appropriate dies away. As he passes through the earth-world mankind loses the gold donkey which eventually stops giving gold. It is better to acquire a healthy power of judgment able to raise itself in freedom above the obscure life of urges and feelings. At first this capacity may seem less valuable than the old power but it gives man wakeful mastery over his own soul-powers.

The cudgel out of the sack is the youthful power of the personality which points to the future. At times it can behave rather uncouthly but it also has the task of making man fight for his freedom. It must fight with the powers that hold sway in the unconscious and would rob the soul of its spirit-heritage. These powers darken man's being but thinking in which the will works strongly has a purifying effect. It gains a sureness of judgment in all real life situations. The fairy-tale tells how the first two brothers are cheated out of their magic gifts and how the third brother with his cudgel restores the gifts to them.

Analysis in terms of the human soul's evolution gives another picture of the fairy-tale. The human being in the time of the sentient-soul still had access to the hidden life-forces; he could acquire the "table set yourself". The age of the intellectual-soul still used the last remains of the inherited clairvoyance; it lived from the golden wisdom of tradition. Modern man, gaining the consciousness-soul as an inner power of freedom, stands at the beginning of quite new capacities, even though they may at first seem insignificant and often crude.

11. Thumbling

The youthful power of the consciousness-soul is still a dwarf in the kingdom of the spirit but it has a powerful urge to conquer. Courage for the world; to explore it, to be submerged in it and to arise intact from it again and again — that is the fundamental characteristic of the Faust-like personality that has appeared since the fifteenth and sixteenth centuries. "Thumbling" is one name for this new force of the self that was born as the son of the tailor. He represents a new will force that

207

tears itself free from the intellectual life of the soul, but not merely as an urge of nature. This new organ is a spiritual force of orientation that begins to awaken in the soul. He appears in the world at first as a revolutionary lacking respect for the old treasures of wisdom. Thumbling throws the king's money out of the window to thieves after stealing into the treasury. Nothing seems safe from him. He hands over the treasures to the robbers and keeps for himself "only one kreuzer" for his travels: he wants to explore the world unburdened. His attitude to life is experimental and for him experience is worth more than tradition.

Not surprisingly this gets him into the cow's dark belly; the world of substance threatens to engulf him. But the power of the human individuality, even though it must live for a time "in the dark" cannot succumb to the darkness of matter in the long run. It wrests itself from the powers of annihilation. Even when Thumbling faces death under the butcher's cleaver, he manages to keep his wits about him. "Danger makes one spry," says the fairy-tale and the consciousness-soul. Formerly one used to say, "danger makes one pray," and that applied fully to the earlier time of the intellectual-soul in its struggle with the world. The youthful self left free by all the protecting powers of the spirit-world, learns to grow strong. It rises again from the depths of matter. The fairy-tale is prophetic anticipating a happy ending for man after all his adventures.

Thumbling seems to bring very little home, only the kreuzer which he took on his wanderings. This plain little coin, on which is stamped the sign of the cross, seems to be a talisman that gives its possessor the power of indestructible life.

The world of the Finnish sagas also knows a thumbling. In the second song of the *Kalevala* when the ancient Vainamoinen prays for help, this thumb-ling comes up out of the sea and fells the giant oak that obscures the beautiful lights of heaven with its branches leaving the earth dark. From the old clair-voyant viewpoint out of which the Finnish myths come, people who give themselves over in dim dreams to the weaving and working of the elements appear in the form of giants. But a being that can compress itself and all its powers into itself is seen as no bigger than a thumb. This is the person who develops powers of thought. Felling the giant oak overcomes the powers of an old race which still live on in warlike urges. Only with the taming of such a racial heritage from Atlan-tean times is it possible for Vainamoinen to imbue the Suomi people with his spirit-powers. This image points to a first powerful infusion of intellectuality into the dimly dreaming folk-soul.

12. *The white snake*

In the "White Snake", the animals of the three kingdoms — under the earth, on the earth, and over the earth — help the seeker of the spirit. He becomes aware, as in the "Three Languages" and the "Queen Bee" of their needs for he can hear "the sighing of the creatures", of which St Paul speaks, because he has eaten of the "White Snake", just as Siegfried heard the language of the birds after the dragon's blood had been sprinkled on his tongue. In the human organism the serpent is bound to the spine. There it is the bearer of those instinctive powers of consciousness connected with the spinal cord. But because our desires have nested there too, the power of temptation is also associated with the serpent. There are, however, still some life-forces which have not been adulterated by the lower urges and remain innocent and wisdom-filled. These are perceived as the white snake.

The human spirit which is awake in the head receives its nourishment from the outside world through sense-perception. But another form of knowledge nourishes the spirit constantly from the realm of dreams. This knowledge is sent up to the head by the nervous system of the spinal cord. That is why the king in the fairy-tale is so "wise". This king holds sway as a higher comprehensive spirit-consciousness within a human nature which still stands in intimate connection with all the kingdoms of creation. The king is inspired out of a cosmic wisdom. But this process which rejuvenates him daily is hidden from ordinary consciousness. Whoever begins to uncover the snake will experience a wisdom which was intended to work only instinctively. It is decisive how he behaves towards these new faculties. If he enters into a moral relationship with that wisdom of worlds which is revealing itself then his path will be blessed, otherwise the supersensory to which he has found access will destroy him.

13. Hats and caps

Hats and caps give people the feeling of being shut in their heads. When a man removes his hat in greeting, he gives up his self-assertion, opens himself for something above and assumes an attitude of reverence. Thus, for example, the cap which shuts off the human self from above plays a part in the story of the "Star Talers". The cap is the first piece of clothing the child has to give up when she goes out into the world. All the earthly thought-forms which close our heads to the world-light and hold us fast in our own world have to be shed if the soul is to raise itself to the spirit. The "Goose Girl" conjures up the wind which blows cheeky Conrad's hat away, and in "Cinderella" a hazel branch brushes the hat off the head of the father who is

[handwritten annotations in top margin: "ng hood → little red riding hood, form of modesty"]

hurrying home. Each time a spirit-power is indicated which pushes back the brain-bound intellect in order to take its place, for only then can the human being become receptive again to the wisdom-filled world thoughts. Anyone who has fallen too much in love with his own little red cap will hardly get away from his personal concerns. He is so proud of his own ideas that he cannot receive higher illumination, resisting any incursion of the grace of the Holy Spirit. The gardener's boy in "Iron Hans", who in order to conceal his golden hair will not doff his hat, represents a different element. His is an attitude of a higher modesty, for the boy wishes to cultivate the powers of the earthly personality and earthly thinking until they are fully ripe. Until then he must wear his "hat" and keep his golden hair hidden. He will not reveal what he already possesses of hidden spirit-light until he has achieved full mastery of the earthly by means of the spirit. That was particularly an ideal of Rosicrucian initiation.

14. The mystery of "fourteen years"

In "Faithful Ferdinand and Faithless Ferdinand" a child is born to two poor people who cannot find a godfather for him. A poor man meets the father and offers to be godfather. In church the mysterious stranger gives the boy the name Faithful Ferdinand, and as a christening gift leaves him a key which is to be kept safe until the boy's fourteenth year. Then the boy is to go out over the heath where he will find a castle which he can open with the key. Whatever lies within the castle is to be his. Everything happens at the right time. A white horse comes out of the castle and Faithful Ferdinand rides out into the world on it. This horse can talk and gives him advice and after many trials he becomes king.

Whether a person can receive the heavenly powers

of wisdom when he awakens to earthly maturity at fourteen depends upon his destiny. What he brings with him to the earth are the forces of his existence in the spirit before birth. He must learn to take hold of these forces within himself at puberty. The fairy-tale points to the mystery in which a spiritual force is laid in the unconscious at baptism, to be grasped consciously at a later stage (in religion marked by the act of confirmation) and further developed.

Faithful Ferdinand meets Faithless Ferdinand who never leaves him and can read his thoughts. He encourages the king with whom both have taken service to misuse Faithful Ferdinand by setting him impossible tasks. Nevertheless the faithful one, with the help of the white horse, succeeds in carrying them out.

Faithless Ferdinand is an image of the human "double", our lower counterpart which can read our secret thoughts and distort them. Faithful, in the language of fairy-tales, means not breaking the connection with the higher self and always acting in unison with the divine world. Unfaithful is the power of soul which seeks to draw us away from our true mission and make us forget our origin. On crossing the threshold indicated by the fourteen years, the youthful soul can become receptive to the ideal: a cosmic spirit-power (the talking white horse) is imparted to it. But at this time the soul forms a link with dark forces of the earth which make the soul faithless to its true nature; a kind of mirror-person that turns all lofty endeavour into caricature begins to find entry into the soul. This can be seen as a demonic force from the realm of Mephistopheles.

The "Devil with the Three Golden Hairs" also depicts soul-experiences which come upon the young person around the time of earth maturity. Certainly one must be a lucky child for the fortune-teller to prophesy by the cradle that one will marry the king's daughter at fourteen! When this time is reached, the lucky child will be led through experiences which express themselves in the well-known feeling of worldly weariness. In the fairy-tale it takes the form of imaginative experiences which mirror the deep perplexity of our time; indeed the sickness which afflicts our whole human existence. A market fountain, out of which once flowed wine, has dried up; a tree that once bore golden apples has withered; a ferryman can find no-one to relieve him. The lucky child, however, "knows it all". He finds the way into the depths of the life of the soul, into "hell". There he obtains three golden hairs from the devil and finds the answers to his questions. Even from the darkness, which otherwise only weighs down upon souls as a nightmare, man can wring prescient wisdom. For there is a golden wisdom with which one can disentangle brooding thought and overcome all despondency.

15. *Forces which have been held back*

Just as Perceval through his upbringing, and the boy in "Iron Hans" through an inwardly awakening force of freedom, were kept from experiencing convention and intellectual rigidity too soon, "Hefty Hans" tells of a boy whose soul-powers have been held back in a most exceptional way until they ripen with elemental force, producing an urge to action so strong nothing in the world can contain or intimidate it.

Hans, an only child, is born in a remote valley. When he is two years old he and his mother are carried off by robbers to a cave. There, in isolation, he grows up with his mother, who teaches him to read out of an old book on chivalry, until he is seized by an uncontrollable desire to find out where he comes from. He overcomes the robbers, breaks out of the cave and returns with his mother to his father's house. But his father's hut cracks and splinters when he puts down the sack full of treasures he has won. The father is horrified at the strength of the twelve-year-old lad.

Here is a soul approaching maturity that breaks through everything that still holds it to heredity and tradition. Hans goes forth in search of adventure and joins up with two gigantic companions, "Fir Twister" who twists the firs like willow wands to make a rope for his faggots, and "Cliff Smasher", who simply punches off pieces of rock with his fists to make a house. Together with these two, Hans performs deeds that reflect activities in the realm of elemental spirits. Fir Twister and Cliff Smasher are forces that work in wild raging storms and earthquakes. But these giant forces can also unleash themselves with violence within our inner being. In the awakening passion of the young person is revealed that storm-giant, the fir twister, and in a revolutionary onslaught against all that is set and rigid is revealed the demon, the cliff smasher. Young people feel compelled to shake the established order and traditional forms of social life. The maturing person, in so far as he is capable of the elemental experiences of youth, must become acquainted with these two companions but must not let himself be overwhelmed by them.

Even more remarkable is the development of soul depicted in "Hans my Hedgehog". Here we have a soul which has a natural predisposition to remain in early childhood. There are souls which incarnate only with strong "reservations". The fairy-tale here gives an indication: the child is born of old parents who have wanted a child for a long time. The child refuses his mother's breast. The story tells that he could not drink from his mother because he would have pricked her with his quills, for Hans is half hedgehog.

For eight years the hedgehog child lies curled up behind the stove; only after that does his inner world begin to stir, though now he wants to go his own way. He cuts himself off from his surroundings and withdraws into his dream-world. The boy in "Iron Hans" also escapes from his parents when he is eight years old and gazes into the fairy-tale gold-fountain. Hans my Hedgehog asks his father for a set of bagpipes, for his soul is full of music, and for a cock to be shod, so that he can ride away and never be seen again. His parents do not understand him, for in human terms he is an "ungifted" child. They cannot be proud of him. Seen from the supersensory, he has a disposition of soul which cannot take hold of the physical body in the "normal" way; it seems bristly, like a hedgehog with quills. But because of this he can develop an inner life of outstanding power and richness. Hans my Hedgehog has melody in himself. He is a lord in the kingdom of dreams, a king of inner worlds. One day he finds his princess and makes his fortune. Then he sheds his hedgehog skin, for now he has reached the point where he can incarnate completely. This soul has rescued his childhood forces and carried them on into later life, forces which "normal" or precocious children use up all too quickly.

The tale of the "Donkey", has a similar theme. The donkey is born to a king, and despite his obvious handicaps learns to play the lute with a famous master. He goes out into the world, and by the power of his music gains entry to a royal palace and the heart of the king's daughter; when he marries her he is able to cast off his donkey-skin.

The fairy-tales have a warm regard for those who have remained childlike — the simple ones. "Hans in

Luck" serves his master for seven years and receives a lump of gold as big as his head. What he has acquired is pure head-knowledge. He feels it as a burden on his life's journey and tries to get rid of it as soon as possible for he is on the way "home to mother". Hans is one of those happy people who cannot lug along what they have learnt and experienced as ballast in their souls, but know how to transform it into formative forces. Finally he receives a heavy grindstone in exchange from a scissors-grinder and rejoices as it drops into a well.

It is into the waters of Lethe that Hans casts his heavy load and the same thing happens to us every night when we go to sleep. All that we have experienced and learned by day sinks into the unconscious, but there it bears fruit for only what we can forget can be transformed into abilities and become instinctive power. We would be able to capture this passing over of the images of our waking-life into the realm of the forgotten if we could experience in waking dreams the moment of going to sleep. First comes the condition in which we lose control of our thoughts. The thoughts fly away: Hans gallops off on the horse, the horse storms away with him, Hans cannot guide the horse properly, and finally it throws him. He exchanges the horse for a cow, the cow for a pig, the pig for a goose, and the goose for the heavy stone which he is happy to see sink in the well. Now he can go back to his mother. He finds the source of the rejuvenation of life. Usually such people are laughed at, yet there are things which appear to the earthly intellect as folly, which can be wisdom before God.

16. The kingdom of the dead

Much may be learned from the way in which fairy-tales speak of the world of the dead. In "Cinderella" the dead mother becomes a source of inspiration for the soul seeking and striving for the spirit. The pictorial language, however, allows a duality. For the mystic "the mother's grave" is an imagination for the ground of one's own soul, but for direct religious experience it can be the real link with the dead mother whom the orphaned girl experiences as her soul's guide and the protector of her destiny.

This story shows those mystical stages whereby the soul can receive its star-raiment from the cosmos. Acts of self-negation are required. The girl must give up sheaths of soul, powers acquired upon earth. Only when complete emptiness has been achieved, a state familiar to the mystics of the Middle Ages, can the supersensory world and its revelations pour in. Here is indicated a condition of soul which leads beyond imagination (the living picture-consciousness); it calls for an extinguishing of the imaginative experiences. Whereas in the formation of images our conceptual faculty still plays a part, the next higher stage of cognition is experienced as receiving pure grace. Rudolf Steiner calls it "inspiration". The consciousness into which the soul grows after death, when the spiritual cosmos begins to grace it with its powers, is fundamentally the same. There too "the empty consciousness" appears as soon as the pictures of earth-life and the desires connected with it have passed away. Only the consciousness "that has become empty" can receive star-grace. Therefore one can regard the fairy-tale of the "Star Talers" as indicating the way of the soul after death and relate it in detail to the stages that it goes through.

The fairy-tale "Mother Holle" is similar. Here too experiences of the mystical path are expressed in fairy-tale pictures. At the same time they reflect most exactly the mysteries of transformation of life after death.

The spindle slips from the girl's hands while she is sitting at the well. She jumps in after it, loses consciousness, and wakes in a lovely meadow. She comes to an oven in which the loaves are fully baked, and to an apple tree on which the fruit is ripe. Obediently she does what she is asked: she takes the bread out of the oven, and shakes the apples from the tree. In this picture of harvesting, an early period of the time after death is accurately portrayed. It is as if all our earthly experiences come to meet us again in reverse order, and in the light of a higher world undergo a kind of after-ripening. They become food for the journey through the spirit: bread and fruit in the kingdom of the dead.

The meeting with the powers of death is represented by the girl's arrival at the house of Mother Holle, whose big teeth frighten the girl. This picture of the teeth points to ossifying powers. Here the girl must set to work. When she shakes the feather-bed it snows on earth. The soul begins to live and weave in mysterious processes that take place in the land of spirit. One can only compare them with the wonderful, pure process of crystallization whereby snow-flakes are formed. Here the spiritual is condensed in the most delicate way to material existence. For the dead it is bliss to take part in such activity and thereby prepare for a new earth-existence, until there begins to awaken longing for the earth however bad life on earth may have been. Mother Holle willingly releases the industrious girl when she wishes to return to earth. She gives her back the spindle, which she needs to take up again the broken-off thread of her life. She leads her to the door from which golden rain showers on the maiden. Henceforth on earth she will be called the "golden maiden" whereas the lazy daughter presents the opposite in every detail and must return through a shower of pitch. This is a soul who in her new life will have ill luck. Her destiny will not be woven through with wisdom and will be unharmonious, for in her former life she wantonly threw her spindle into the well. She cannot develop any interest for her life's fruits, and in Mother Holle's realm of pure crystallizing wisdom she prepares for her future existence without love. She lacks faithfulness to the earth and has no love for human duties. Such a soul must enter a new life with a darkened disposition.

The fairy-tales depict the laws of transformation and hint at the mysteries of recurring earth-lives and the compensatory working of destiny (karma). These latter teachings were suppressed in the Middle Ages by Christian dogma but survived in the wisdom of the mystics.

The fairy-tale "Godfather Death" points clearly to this same mystery of life and death. The youth who has Death himself as godfather (this ancient motif has come down to us in several variations) receives from him the gift of being able to heal all sicknesses. For that he is given a wonderful herb. He may use his knowledge only when Death shows himself at the head, but never the foot of the patient. This signifies an initiation into the mysteries of the art of healing. The initiate-doctor may never heal "against destiny". His clairvoyant vision beholds the power of death in the body of the patient. He is well aware that death-forces are always operative in man's being and that they reside in the ossifying processes which work through the body's organization downward, whereas the building-up processes, which are the source of all healing effects, work through the body upward. When Death stands at the head of the bed all is in order, but when he stands at the foot, this means he has taken hold of the complete organism of the patient who becomes marked for death. This law must be respected by the initiate. The fairy-tale tells now how the doctor comes under the temptation to heal "against fate" and how this rebounds against him. Death leads him into a cave where he sees the life-lights of people — long ones, half-burned down, and very small ones. Godfather Death shows him his own, which to his horror is tiny. All his pleading that his godfather light him a new, long candle is in vain. Death himself cannot do this. "First one must go out before a new one can be lit," the godfather says. The inexorability of death, the sacro-sanct nature of the laws of existence, but also the implication of the mystery whereby the light of life shall sometime be kindled in hidden depths to new life, all this the fairy-tale seeks to show us in its pictures.

17. The hidden picture

The motif from "Faithful John" is also touched on in the "White Bride and the Black Bride" where the guardian of the picture is Raynald, which means adviser. He is the king's coachman and has painted the picture of his sister who is pure and beautiful as the sun. He hangs it secretly in his room but a courtier tells the king who orders it to be brought to him. There-upon he falls mortally in love with her and orders Raynald to fetch his sister for his bride. But Raynald, bewitched by the wicked stepmother, delivers the stepsister, who is "as black as night and as ugly as sin". The disappointed king has Raynald cast into a snake pit.

That is the destiny of an initiate. He who knows, hides the picture of the "white bride". He is the guardian of the pure archetype of man. When, however, the seeker after knowledge requires it, the initiate must do him the service of acquiring the "bride". Iron Heinrich in the "Frog King" is also a coachman, and in the *Bhagavadgita* it is also a charioteer who initiates King Arjuna; in the charioteer, however, the divine Krishna reveals himself.

The seeker of wisdom, when the mediator of higher cognition passes on knowledge to him, is disappointed because he first becomes acquainted with the lower form of wisdom: intellectual knowledge. He must learn that he has to release the pure form of wisdom from the spell of misshapenness. When, however, it is made to resemble the picture, Raynald is welcomed back. Having overcome the lower form of knowledge it is possible to acknowledge again the mediator of higher wisdom.

One of the best known versions of this theme is the Egyptian legend of the "Veiled Picture at Sais". Viewing the goddess, the youth falls senseless before the picture which "Faithful John" has to show him. For the legend says: "No mortal may lift her veil and go unpunished." To this warning Novalis in his "Disciples at Sais" gave the only answer worthy of mankind: "We must then seek to become immortal."

17

Fairy-tales around the world

1. Russian fairy-tales

The peoples of the earth are called upon to know each other, so they can work together in understanding and mutual appreciation within the organism of mankind. Where they fail to do so they will confront each other violently. Even this leads to knowledge of one another but in a painful way and the pictures they gain of one another are often distorted by fear. Much will have to happen before the folk-souls of Europe learn to see each other in a pure light and truly come to understand one another.

Fairy-tales, coming from old folklore, are the most immediate revelation of the folk-soul and of all that dreams and yearns within its depths — not only the high ideals active within it but also the unfulfilled urges and unredeemed violence rumbling in the depths.

In the great collection of fairy-tales made by Afanas'ev* in the middle of the last century the figure of "Ivan" — who is of course "John" — comes to the fore. He is a lovable, and at times laughable, character but he has remarkable traits, and behind him there

---

* See *Russian Fairy Tales* collected by Aleksandr Afanas'ev. Panther Books, New York 1975.

begins to shine what we might call a Johannine spiritual endeavour.

Afanas'ev was still imbued with that reverence for folk tradition which leaves the cadence and style of the old fairy-tales as far as possible untouched: he has a feeling for their inner truth and for the spiritual background of the images. He says: "People did not just invent it all: they spoke of what they believed, and therefore in speaking of the supersensory they did not let imagination run riot and lose itself in a world full of grotesque mental images."

From the great variety of these fairy-tales we can draw together all the traits of character which belong to the archetypal figure of the Russian seeker after the spirit. For Ivan is the seeker after wisdom and beauty, after "Vasilisa, the Wise", and "Vasilisa the Beautiful", the king's daughter who is held prisoner or who waits "beyond thrice nine kingdoms" for her suitor. She represents the shining Virgin Sophia — the wisdom-soul of mankind, entrusted to the guardianship of St John, the beloved disciple of the Lord. John stands as leader in the evolution of Christian mankind, preparing souls for the age of the Holy Spirit in which the Russian people will have a leading task.

Ivan, or the king's son "John", appears often as the youngest of three sons: he is usually the simpleton, as in many German fairy-tales. Because of his heart-forces he proves himself fit for the hardest tasks. Sometimes indeed it is stressed that his development has been retarded so that it could break through all the more powerfully at a later time. In the fairy-tale "I Do Not Know", Ivan, the peasant's son, has turned thirty-three and still cannot walk. His parents keep on praying to God to give their son healthy feet. After a church service a beggar comes to their hut and begs for alms. Ivan would like to give him some, but cannot rise from the spot. "Stand up and give me alms. your feet are healed," says the beggar. At once Ivan rises and invites the beggar into the hut to be his guest. The beggar, however, does not drink the honey-mead which the young man offers him but requires him to drain the vessel himself. Whereupon Ivan is filled with great strength.

Here, we are presented with a spiritual awakening, such as can take place around the thirty-third year through the Christ-forces. When Ivan sets forth upon his travels into the world, he finds the hero-steed with smoking ears and flaming nostrils. The horse tells Ivan it has been waiting for him with all its strength for thirty-three years. It is exactly as old as himself. It is his own held-back spirit-power, a fiery intelligence that carries him high above forests, mountains and valleys and leads him to the famous fairy-tale goals.

Often when the king's son comes into a foreign kingdom he is asked: "Did you come here of your own free will or by force?" Here one recognizes the seeker after the worlds of spirit, for he travels ways of soul that can be travelled only in inmost freedom. No outside force compels him. When by spiritual initiative high resolves are to be taken, they will be affected by no inner compulsion arising from habit or from the region of desire in the body-bound human being.

"Purely of my own free will I came here," answers Ivan. "I seek my mother, Queen Anastasia with the golden tresses. A storm-wind stole her out of our garden ..." A human nature shaken by the storms of passion has lost access to the original wisdom that once shone in the mother-depths of the soul. The name Anastasia means "Easterlike": in it lies that close and deep relationship of the Russian soul to the Easter mystery, the knowledge of the resurrection of the spirit which has been lost to mankind.

Three kingdoms must be passed through to win her again; the copper, the silver, and the gold. From ancient traditions we know the teaching of the three ages of the world, the gold, silver and bronze (or copper) which have preceded our own. Hesiod described them for the Greeks. In Goethe's fairy-tale of the "Green Snake and the Beautiful Lily" the three kings, who await their awakening from enchantment in the underground temple, are also characterized as the golden, the silver and the bronze.

The human being, if he is to awaken to his true existence and enter upon his highest dignity, must rediscover the primal world-wisdom and world-forces that belonged to man in paradise. To the seeker after the lost mother these forces reveal themselves as three kingdoms that lie in the depths of the soul awaiting release from their enchantment. A voice speaks to Ivan: "Never yet have I seen the Russian spirit with my eyes, never yet have I heard him with my ears, but now the Russian spirit appears before my eyes." Thus Ivan, the king's son is greeted. Thus the Russian spirit presses on irresistibly to those spheres in which there dwells beauty and wisdom, the Virgin Sophia who is waiting to be wedded to the seeking human spirit. Eventually the Russian spirit will reveal itself in all its depth and show what it can mean to the world once it assumes its true character.

"They were married and gave a banquet for the whole world," we are told in the fairy-tale of "Ivan, Son of the Cow" who won the Tsarevna with the golden hair. This is a power of soul that would like to be sister to the world. It has still to go through many trials, but will at some time ripen to its illumination in the spirit.

Certainly it will first have to face up to the powers of death: these appear in the picture of the "undying skeleton". When the undying skeleton breaks the twelve iron chains forged round it, seizes "Mary, the sea's daughter" and cuts up Ivan, the king's son, into tiny bits, this signifies the human spirit's transit through the age of materialistic thought-forms and of unleashed technology. But all the fairy-tales know how to bring the spirit back to life. They know the water of life and its magic power that can reawaken the king's son who was cut to pieces. They know too, the mystery of how that which has been won in the spirit can be brought gradually into earth reality. The fairy-story, the "Sea King and Vasilisa the Wise" tells how Ivan, after the royal wedding with Vasilisa, sets off on a journey into "Holy Russia". Transformations are depicted. In the fairy-tale pictures are reflected stages of an apocalyptic, Christian evolution. Unrecognized and in deep humility, Sophia, the Radiant Beauty, steps into "Holy Russia". She takes service with a baker's wife in order to help bake bread for the altar. This signifies that Sophia imparts her all-ensouling forces to the stream of consecration that goes through the holy service at the altar. They come to remind the king's son of his holy union with the "Wise". It is the hour of the doves; the coming of the age of spirit illumination towards which Johannine Christianity is striving and for which all true fairy-tale heroes fight, suffer and win victories.

Hard indeed the roads that the Russian folk-soul is destined to travel. In Russia too, the story of the "Girl without Hands" is told. Fundamentally it is similar to the German fairy-tale but the Russian version makes the mystery of the child central. The woman without hands gives birth to a son: "His arms up to the elbows were in gold, stars twinkled on his hips, the bright moon on his brow and the golden sun upon his heart."

Here, clearly, a supersensory birth graced by the

227

forces of the whole cosmos is represented. When the man casts out his wife, the babe is bound to the poor mother's breast and she is sent away. She bends down over a well because she is thirsty, and the star-child slips away and sinks into the water. The mother walks helplessly round the edge of the well. An old man comes and commands her: "Bend down and pull your child out." "Little father, I have no hands, only arms to the elbows." But he again commands her. She stretches her arms down into the well and hands grow again. She is able to draw her child out of the depths.

Is not this the destiny of the Russian soul? It is condemned to impotence and may only bear its star-mystery in its heart — a holy hope of the future. This soul has had to let the divine child sink and now it stands in despair before the Well of Lethe. But there is a power of yearning so strong that it can bring about the miracle. Those who have knowledge say: the arms will grow, spirit-arms that will lift up the star-child out of the depths. Then he will be shown to the world. For the soul of the Russian, filled with the light of Christ, shall in future times proclaim the message of the higher, cosmic self. Man, as a being in whom all the heavens created an image of themselves, will understand himself. And by taking hold of himself with understanding he will vanquish the power of darkness.

2. Fairy-Tales from Grisons

In the course of European history the Swiss canton Grisons (Graubünden) has become in many ways the intersection of important currents. First we should note the original heritage of the old Rhaetians, who in their mountain valleys were able to preserve a natural clairvoyance for a long time. For them, meetings with elemental beings were commonplace. Through the influence of the Alemannic element thrusting down from the north, rich cultural traditions were implanted deep in the souls of these peoples. Grisons also had a connection with French culture in the seventeenth century and the continuous influence of Italian culture, particularly in the Engadine. This explains why the collectors of Grisons fairy-tales were able at a comparatively late date to bring in such a rich and varied harvest.

The lofty world of high mountain peaks of the Grisons finds a reflection in its fairy-tales. The "Three Winds" describes the dialogue of the soul with three guardians of inner development whom we often meet in the stories as the trinity of the soul's powers. A youth is placed by his parents in the care of an old hermit to save him from falling into the power of the "Lord with the Green Coat". The devil often appears in the form of a green-jacketed man. The hermit now teaches the boy to read in a book "that was as old as Methuselah" and leads him to the place where two roads make a cross. For a long time the boy, faithfully obeying the commands of his teacher and master, reads the book until a mighty eagle seizes him in its talons and carries him off high into the air. But because the boy goes on calmly reading the book the eagle has to let go of him. The fairy-tale affirms: "And really and truly he came down to earth on the top of the Julier Pass," indicating experiences of the spirit.

The hermit points the way towards living in meditation, and the description of the youth hearing a sound "as of a host of witches" just before the eagle carries him off, illustrates wonderfully the transition that lifts the soul out of meditation into the consciousness that is free of the body.

The youth begins his initiation after a year-long

preparation, far from everyday affairs, on top of the Julier Pass. He finds three benevolent fairies who dwell in a glorious palace of clearest crystal. They take on his development and he is allowed to enjoy a wonderful relationship with them. When, however, he comes to the time when his beard begins to grow, he falls in love with the most beautiful fairy. They prepare for the wedding. But now the obstacles of life begin to take effect and threaten to entangle him in the circle of his parents and earthly inclinations when he has to go down again into the valley. Only after a difficult spirit-search and many adventures does the youth succeed in reaching again the heights of the Julier and finding the entrance to the crystal palace to celebrate the longed-for wedding.

But the light of Christian mysticism, too, shines into the soul of Grisons. Thus we find the well-known motif of the release from enchantment of the raven-nature most impressively developed in a fairy-tale called the "Raven". It tells of a poor count, who is very anxious about his one single little daughter; the dearest thing he has on earth. One day he goes downcast through the wood, wondering what may become of the child after his death. Then he hears a raven's voice: "Bring me your daughter and I will give you as much gold as you desire." The count leads the maiden into the wood and hands her over to the feathered bridegroom.

It is anxiety for the eternal that moves the seeker after the spirit: in the language of medieval Christianity one would say for "the soul's salvation". The raven tells the maiden that a witch cast a spell upon him when he was a fine-looking youth. So now he, who was once a prince with rich treasures, has to live as a raven in the dark wood.

"Sweet maid," says he, "follow me to my castle. Go into the chapel there. Kneel at the altar for one whole day, weep and pray to God. Fill the jar that stands there ready with your tears, and when I come in the evening sprinkle my feathers with it. But do not let one drop fall to the ground."

In the raven fairy-tale of the "Twelve Brothers", the condition for breaking the spell was seven year's silence; here the condition is more clearly clothed in the language of mystical wisdom, pointing to a schooling of the soul. It takes place in the holiest of holies of man's being, in the abode of the heart, where the soul ripens to sacrifice. In the chapel of the palace the maiden must kneel at the altar for one whole day and pray to God. Powers of atonement must be engendered to effect the transformation of the spiritual part of man's being.

The indications are given in imaginative language and point to powers of concentration. In the evening, when the raven returns, the maiden is to bring the jar filled with her tears and pour it out over his feathers: but no drop is to be spilt. Twice she fails, and the raven says sadly: "If you spill tears for the third time, then I shall have to fly about in the forest for a hundred years."

It is also told of the griffin that only once in a hundred years does he give away one of his golden feathers. Not every day is someone chosen by the spirit. In the course of human evolution the impulses of supersensory life appear at rhythmical intervals. Therefore it is of the greatest importance not to let the moment of grace slip by. The jar filled with tears represents the fruits of contemplation which must be borne over the threshold of going to sleep. What has been experienced in the depths of feeling must be united with that part of our being which by day leads a shadow-existence. During waking hours our powers of thought lose themselves in the sense-world. But when they return to the inmost part of our being we should give them back to the life of the spirit. They rejoice in their resurrection when they have been brought to life again by the heart's power of sacrifice, but this requires a capacity for inmost recollection that has to be acquired by practice.

The story emphasizes the mystical nature of the wedding between the maiden and the prince who is indebted to her for his release. The story ends: "I waited at table, and when I dropped the soup they gave me a kick which sent me flying right here." This is not just any wedding but one which can be celebrated everywhere and in every soul once the inner conditions for it have been set up. For it is that "Royal Wedding" to which all are invited who have heard the call. At this wedding the lower self must render proper service to the higher self. For the earthly person it is difficult to keep awake and not let those swiftly fleeting experiences slip away when he needs to bring their fairy-tale splendour safely over into everyday consciousness. The narrator feels all too keenly the inadequacy of his own spiritual maturity: and so he speaks of his own clumsiness at the wedding and the kick which so rudely sends him back into everyday consciousness. But the humour indicates a healthy self-knowledge. In him, the consciousness of having been chosen accompanies that deep humility to which all genuine self-knowledge will lead the disciple of wisdom.

A similar ending is found in many Grisons fairy-tales. Thus the story-teller of the three miller's sons who made their fortune ends: "As I was just passing through this town, they invited me to the wedding." He is still revelling in the memory of the feast. Then it goes on: "When I had eaten and drunk enough, they told me the story of the three miller's sons. Then a servant took me by the ear and said: "Be off with you and tell other people the story too'."

Again the story-teller avows that he has partaken of such hallowed moments of spiritual experience. But here too we find the drastic manner in which consciousness is brought back into the everyday world. The earthly person has no cause to give himself airs with what he has experienced for he has been dismissed without much ceremony. Nevertheless he feels the obligations laid upon him by such experiences.

The story of the wonderful shining bird which alights on the left shoulder of the wandering youth is humorous, too. It is the bird of inspiration that whispers the wisdom of the fairy-tale into his ear and so is desired of all who see it. The "Golden Goose" in Grimms' fairy-tales is related to this, although it is more elaborate in individual motifs. Here again, it is a question of healing the king's daughter. This time she is not really ill but only very sad. She is the "princess who could not laugh". A son of poor people has heard of her misfortune and also of the king's promise that anyone who can make her laugh shall have her as bride. On his way to the palace he meets an old woman who tells him a beautiful bird will alight on his left shoulder. He must look after the bird and on no account give it away. The bird duly appears. Stopping at an inn, he finds many people anxious to buy the bird, but he refuses. The innkeeper, however, tries to steal the bird while the youth is asleep. He creeps to the youth's bed at midnight to carry off the bird but when he touches it he sticks to its feathers. The same happens to the innkeeper's wife, who tries to free her husband, and to the maid. Each one is stuck fast to the one in front.

Next morning the youth passes through the village

with his bird and those who are stuck to it. The parson, angered at seeing this procession, runs after it but also gets stuck. The same thing happens to the baker's wife when she tries to pull the parson clear. Finally, the procession comes to the palace, and the princess cannot help laughing at the sight. As a reward the youth is allowed to marry her.

The pictures in the fairy-tale seem at first to be lightly woven, but the thought hidden behind them is audacious. It became apparent to those with knowledge that the development of a rigid intellectualism threatened the soul. They felt the one-sided intellectual culture was settling upon souls and laming them and could point to ecclesiastical theology, becoming set in its dogmas, as having a considerable part in this fatal development. Only a wisdom that could be clothed in colourful pictures of the imagination could free the soul of rigidity and give it the experience of spiritual freedom. To be able to laugh is a sign of inner liberation.

The youth who heals the princess's affliction is the seeker after those living forces of the spirit which can lead the soul out of the bonds of a one-sided intellectual development and bring a pictorial experience of the riddles of existence. In the old woman who accosts him he meets the ancient original wisdom. She recognizes in him a chosen one of the spirit, one blessed with imagination. Incorruptible, not exploiting his gift for any other ends, he serves his calling among men and the effects of the bird's inspiration become apparent and spread over to other souls. The narrative describes in part a nocturnal experience. The youth has the gift of being able to tell fairy-tales and sagas. He has been given the power to draw human hearts into the magic circle of his imagination. The pictures that shine with wisdom do not only give fleeting

234

impressions; they penetrate much more deeply than the souls can imagine. They work on in the night. The souls cannot get away from them for while they sleep they are held by the picture's magical power. The souls desire the magic bird and are caught in its spell.

This free way of the spirit that seeks to spread the wisdom of the higher worlds in fairy-tale and saga pictures found its greatest opponents in the established Church. The theologian who kept the spirit imprisoned in dogmas often showed himself as the arch-enemy of those trying to sow their spirit-seed in the language of imagination. We find a picture of this opposition in the fairy-tale with the angry parson trying to free his parishioners. But he too falls under the spell of the inspired story-telling and dances to the soaring spirit's flight.

And so the princess, the abject human soul, laughs with joy to see the soul's release in union with the spirit.

Finally let us select from the wealth of motifs one more characteristic fairy-tale in which the picture sequence is manifestly inspired by esoteric Christianity. We have already commented, in connection with the winter mysteries, on this Grisons fairy-tale, the "Enchanted Prince", which takes as its starting-point the search for the rose that blossoms in the depths of winter. In it, the prince, changed into a snake by a witch, crawls out of the spring while the miller is plucking the beautiful rose for his daughter. To win the rose, one must first free the snake. The purification of the blood, appearing in the picture of the mystical rose, is conditional on the soul becoming acquainted with the forces that still hold sway in the blood. The fairy-tale says the soul must have the courage to light the candle in the night while she is united with her mysterious husband.

Only the light of cognition can release the snake

from enchantment; on everything that is still veiled in the soul's depths it has a liberating effect. But such cognition is at first still clouded by the senses, and the miller's daughter loses her prince in the same way as Psyche in the Greek tale "Eros and Psyche". The light of cognition is not yet sustained by complete composure of heart. It ought only to illuminate, but it also burns, for passion is still mixed with it. The fairy-tale's images of purification show an unmistakably Christian undertone. After the prince and palace have vanished the miller's daughter sees before her only a thorn bush and a pair of iron shoes. She must wander the world until she has worn out the iron shoes. Iron shoes bring the feet right down to the earth, so the soul may not flutter away in spirit-light.

The miller's daughter meets an old woman who advises her to put the shoes in a cowpat so they will rust away. This image from the life of a pastoral people points towards humble earthly service. The brilliance of supersensory light needs the balance of healthy ties with the earth forged firmly through service.

After the poor maid has worn out her iron shoes in this way, she comes to a king's palace and asks for shelter. The queen takes her in and the miller's daughter gives birth to a child. At the same moment a mysterious voice is heard: "The golden lamp and the silver staff! If thy grandmother but knew it, she would wrap thee in golden napkins. If the cocks should not crow and the bells should not ring, I would come to thee!"

The following midnight the queen's maids hear the same words while keeping watch. The queen has all the cocks killed and the bells silenced and keeps watch by the young mother. When the voice at midnight speaks the same words the queen answers: "The cocks do not crow, and the bells do not ring so come to us."

236

And then the miller's daughter's prince, who is also the queen's son, appears, freed from his enchantment. The wedding can now be celebrated.

The exalted being who announces his coming so mysteriously at midnight can reveal himself only in the deepest silence. When the voices of the day are hushed this being can wake to life. The solemn words that preface his appearance testify that something most holy will impart itself to the soul. Nothing of the snake's nature is left clinging to him; he has cast off the fetters of the senses.

This being announces himself to the soul when the royal child is born. This son is the fruit of the mysterious relationship the girl has with the enchanted prince. The soul has become creative, although it could receive the seed of this young kingly power only from hidden realms. It could, however, ripen within the girl while she willingly practised "standing with iron shoes in warm cowpats". The inspiration from above must be nourished with the earth's pristine forces, and these can be acquired only by faithfulness to the things of every day. The tale of "Eros and Psyche" describes how the soul becomes fit through purification to partake of the divine life. She is carried up to Olympus. But the Grisons fairy-tale shows it is necessary to develop within the inner being of the soul a seed of creative life, and that this new life is the deepest expression of a personality united with the earth.

The mysterious voice promises the royal child "the golden lamp and the silver staff". Whoever can call the golden lamp his own knows the grace of illumination that can reveal the hidden. Whoever possesses the shepherd's silver staff has a king's sceptre and by its gentle magic knows how to direct the soul's urges. The child, born at midnight, will be a ruler in the kingdom of the beautiful for beauty is the gentle reflection of wisdom.

But who in this fairy-tale is the exalted consecrator? He is the redeemed snake. Lucifer is transformed into the Genius of Wisdom and Beauty when the soul woos the mystery of the rose that blossoms only in the depths of winter in an obscure place. Through the pristine power of a pastoral people the fairy-tale heroine attains the exalted goal which she has chosen in freedom.

3. Fairy-tales from Gascony

Gascony, in the South of France, is a land of a former high spiritual culture. It is the homeland of the Cathars in whom a Christianity illuminated by Manichaean wisdom flowered until it was extinguished by the Church of Rome in the gruesome wars against them. Through the songs of the troubadours something of this high culture was carried and in the simple garb of the fairy-tale it passed on into the folk-mind.

Many cultural influences find a reflection in these fairy-tales. The Celtic influence is found in their intimacy with the elemental spirits. Centuries of Graeco-Roman cultural life finds expression in motifs related to the sagas of Oedipus and Odysseus. There is also the influence of the Visigoths — who founded the kingdom of Toulouse and whose nobility patronized the minnesinger culture — which, united with the wisdom of the Cathars, gives these fairy-tales their particular ethos.

Closely related to the "Griffin" is the fairy-tale of the "Three Oranges". Here it is made even clearer that we have to do with the golden fruit of the Hesperides, which hide within them the mystery of the Tree of Life, the miraculous rejuvenation of man's being. The best doctor in Montpellier says to the king: "Your daughter will regain her health, but the means of healing her is not to be found here; it is far, far away in the land of the oranges. In that land stands a beautiful garden where it neither snows nor freezes. In this garden stands an orange tree, strewn with white blossom, and in it seven hundred nightingales sing day and night. On the orange tree are growing nine gold-red oranges. Sire, send but one young man thither to pick three oranges and bring them hither. After your daughter has eaten the first, she will rise from her bed. After the second, she will be more beautiful and healthier than she has ever been. After the third orange, she will say: "I shall have neither peace nor rest until I have married the young man who has brought me the three oranges'."

The realm of the elements is described by the story-tellers partly from their own vision: "As true as we all shall die, I speak only of that which I know myself, and moreover I could prove without trouble all that I present." This is the testimony of a story-teller who can still describe precisely the life-habits of the "little people". Then we are told these beings go harvesting once a year on New Year's Eve. This points to that mystery of deep winter when the Spirit of the Earth comes to its brightest waking in the Holy Nights and the elemental beings gather in the fruits of the earth for the life of the coming year.

In another fairy-tale the hero makes his way into an enchanted castle. When midnight strikes he finds himself in the midst of the little creatures. Strange beings suddenly fall down the chimney piece by piece: legs, hands and heads singly — but finally they fit together like the parts of a machine, and in soulless activity they dance, singing the same words rhyth-mically. They count out the days from Monday to

Friday — the working days; they do not know Satur-
day and Sunday, the hallowed days of the Old and
New Covenant. They confess that the first five days are
"for bodies without souls". But these beings long for
someone who can make the whole week holy. The hero
has penetrated into a realm of subnature from which
the soul-destroying powers of technology rise up.
There he becomes aware of busy beings who are
pressing to enter the service of man in order to receive
from him their ensoulment, their Christianization,
which can come about only by the hallowing from
Sunday of the working week.

The same youth, who has grown up an orphan and
herdsman in a village in the South of France, can also
make his way into a realm of supernature. In a
deserted chapel at night he finds the world of the dead
and it is granted to him to receive the altar sacrament
for the first time from the hands of a priest who has
died and who now celebrates mass. The priest discovers a golden lily stamped on the youth's tongue: a
sign that he is of royal French blood.

But these fairy-tales do not speak of the outward
kingdom; the king represents nobility of spirit, whose
fire the troubadours felt coursing through their veins.
When the youth returns from the world of the dead,
he finds the old Maltese sword behind the altar of the
chapel. With this sword he will at some time accomplish the deed of liberation for it will cut through the
wind beneath whose breath a mighty magician holds
himself hidden.

The sword which is received from the altar is the
power of the Word itself. This spirit-sword cuts
through the wind showing itself master over the forces
of breathing. The youth with the golden lily on his
tongue relies upon the magic of the Word, a consecrated power of speech. He who was known before as a

bastard is now installed in his royal dignity. He is, as the fairy-tale calls him, "the king's true son". In such fairy-tales the mission of poetry, the holy service of the Word, is celebrated. As a last echo of the high culture of the troubadour it vibrates in the hearts of the people. The lyrical note that gives the German fairy-tales their magic mood and speaks so distinctively to the child's heart is not to be found here. It is replaced by the ballad tone.

The style of these fairy-tales is so resolute that it immediately captures the reader. He is carried along by the rhythm of the hero's steps — a rhythm that brooks no obstacle once a high objective is sighted. Thus in the "Golden Dragoon", the count's son comes on his flying horse through the clouds as swift as lightning, in the full spirit-power of a warrior of Michael. He rescues "the damsel in the white robe" from her grievous plight as Perceval frees Blanchefleur. He forces the Lord of Night to the ground. This lord has carried off the dragoon's bride and is holding her under a magic spell. When vanquished he says: "You are stronger than I, yet you cannot kill me. It is written that I shall live until the last judgment, but then I shall arise no more."

Until the end of the earth man will need this power of darkness as his opponent. This is Manichaean thinking that lived in Catharism. Only by coming constantly to grips with that power can the highest good be achieved. So we see simple figures helping the soul in its struggle. Such a figure is the beggar with the long white beard in the fairy-tale of the "Louse". He is called "Jack o' the Woods" and recalls one of the "bonhomme", as the bearer of the spirit in the Cathar communities was called. He appears before the miller's daughter and promises her a fine young suitor.

241

But his opponent, "the gold-spitter", is already there. This ragamuffin, two ells high and as black as the inside of a chimney, comes up to her threateningly and boasts of his might, for he has turned her betrothed into a louse. She will have to be married to a louse unless she can answer three riddles. She answers the riddles trusting the voice of the louse who has crawled into her ear. The louse can see through the evil one's wiles. At the critical moment he crawls into the mouth of the miller's daughter and answers for her, breaking the spell of the satanic power.

The last scenes are delightful. The youth is released from the spell, and Jack o' the Woods reappears to advise the mill folk to cudgel the gold-spitter until he has spat out all the gold pieces he has swallowed. Now the miller's daughter and the youth are rich and can celebrate their wedding. That means that the soul finds its higher being, the spirit which at first comes to it in a quite insignificant guise but whose voice is able to encourage the human heart and speak for the soul in its trials. Only in grappling with the power of life does the soul realize its true self. Without having struggled with evil it would never have been able to acquire that wealth of experience which displays itself as wisdom-gold. Such fairy-tales that could speak of the meaning of evil and of dealing with it were spread abroad by the bonhommes within the Cathar communities in the twelfth and thirteenth centuries.

In these southern French fairy-tales the moral world-order is led to victory in an heroic manner. In the most striking fashion this is accomplished in the fairy-tale of the "Singing Sea, the Dancing Apple, and the Prophesying Bird". In this story the wicked queen is convicted of her evil deeds. The young king, her son, sentences her to a hundred lashes and then execution. But because the people say "the son may not condemn his mother to death," the king takes upon himself the punishment. He has himself bound to a stake and flogged. When the executioner unbinds him: "He was in such a sorry state that everyone felt pity for him. But he did not weep, for a man may not weep, especially when he is the ruler and when he stands before his people." But when the executioner's sword shatters three times on the kings neck, it is apparent that divine justice has been done and no further sacrifice is required.

The true fairy-tale hero appears as a youth in the fairy-tale of the "Man in all Colours". He is the youngest of a poor woodcutter's seven sons. Before sending him out into the world his father gives him as a parting gift a robe made up of all the colours, while each of the elder brothers receives a gold piece. The father consoles him for being able to give him only the patchwork garment. Yet one feels that in this gift, though it leaves the human being outwardly poor, there lies a hidden power similar to that of Joseph's coat of many colours which he received from his father, Jacob, and which distinguished him from his brothers. For Joseph became thereby the "dreamer". It is a soul-garment which endows its owner with dream powers. It gives him the power of imagination whereby he is able to know the secrets of the inner life. He can now step forth on the road to initiation.

The fairy-tale of the "Veiled One" is also stirring. Someone who has gone astray but having realized his error treads the path of atonement, can become a great helper of men. Unrecognized, he performs deeds that affect the life of the people. As a last act of healing he saves his people from the black death. But to achieve this he has first to pluck the golden flower on an island in the sea: "The balsam flower that sings like a nightingale." It is the power of poetry, which as a world-illuminating force can heal human souls from that black pestilence which must overtake them if they lose their connection with the world of the spirit and are thus exposed to the death of the soul.

4. Nordic fairy-tales

In the Nordic fairy-tale tradition, the elemental world appears in a more monstrous guise. Gigantic trolls everywhere oppose the seeker after the spirit. Atavistic faculties kindled in human souls by the powerful nature-forces of Scandinavia are a real danger for these people. In the fairy-tale of "Peer Gynt", it is mountain experiences which menace the intrepid huntsman from without and within. "The Great Bent One" who opposes him is a troll who rises up both from the surroundings and from his own inner life. Chaotic forces play through the imaginative world of the Nordic fairy-tales. They threaten to stifle the awakening self in its freedom. Everywhere this self is called upon to struggle.

The most impressive picture of these gigantic powers is in the fairy-tale of the "Golden Castle that Hung in the Air". The fight with the many-headed trolls, the taming of the dragon and the rescue of the three maidens from the enchanted castle are motifs that give the fairy-tale a Michaelic character. The basic theme of this Nordic fairy-tale world might be called "the self that fights its way to freedom". In this fairy-tale the wise donkey who counsels and encourages the youth is a particularly attractive figure. When the mountain troll leads the hero, Ashpeter, into his stable, Ashpeter does not choose a gold or silver horse, but the little grey donkey. Ashpeter is a male Cinderella (Ashputtle): he remains modestly on the borders of the earthly world. The donkey gives him the power which we can gain by being awake in our bodies. The donkey's rider does not allow himself to be carried away by the driving-force of the horse, be it noble or base, for the donkey is of a gentler nature. Level-headedness guides the spirit-seeker who undertakes his heroic journey on his back. Christ himself rode on an ass into Jerusalem to reveal his kingdom of the spirit.

By nature, Nordic man may have an inclination towards excess. Therein lies the scale of his possibilities but also his vulnerability. Think of the figures of Brand and Peer Gynt; one can include also the visions of such a man as Emmanuel Swedenborg which are boundless and in a certain sense unclarified. The fairy-tale warns Peer Gynt: Anyone who forthwith seizes the gold or the silver horse can at best become only a day-dreamer or a visionary. He is always in danger of becoming a spiritual fraud. But anyone who, like Ashpeter, recognizes that the horses are too big and keeps strictly to the calm forces of thinking, however insignificant they may appear to be at first, will learn to overcome the chaos of the soul. These forces alone can clarify his spirit and help him see the high objectives of the spirit light up before him. They will steady his mind when it feels itself thrown off balance by the nightmare of the elemental powers. In this regard the conversation between the donkey and Ashpeter as they approach one of the great objectives and the donkey draws his rider's attention to the corresponding dangers, is relevant. "I think I am afraid," says the lad. "Oh, who should be afraid?" laughs the donkey, who then gives appropriate advice on coping with the approaching powers. In the end the donkey has to be beheaded. Otherwise man would not be able to overcome his animal nature and become a human power.

Inspiring wisdom still works as an instinctive soul-force in the spirit-seeker. But it passes over into the measured clarity of thinking. It induces inner freedom in thinking and in action. All mediumistic conditions or visionary experiences, in so far as they arise out of an old heritage of folk-nature, are overcome by the true spirit-seeker; only he must know how to match daring with wakeful level-headedness.

5. African fairy-tales

The memory of the cosmic origin of our being lives in the wisdom of all myths and sagas, including those of Africa. Kimanaueze's son, so tells an African fairy-story, is to marry. But he will take no girl of the earth: "If I must marry, I will marry only a daughter of the Lord Sun and Lady Moon." The people shake their heads, for who could climb up to the sky? The youth, however, writes a marriage application to the Sun-Father and gives it to the frog. The daughters of the sky come down to earth on cobwebs in order to draw water from a well and the frog slips into a water-pot so he can carry the letter up to the sky.

Kimanaueze's son knows of his eternal being that has remained in the heights of light. He wishes to find this eternal being and reunite himself with cosmic consciousness. In the "Frog King", the frog retrieves the lost ball from the well and in the African fairy-tale, too, the frog represents an old stage in the development of the soul: a memory of ancient times when the sun-forces were still potent in the earth. Delicate cobwebs still unite the earth today with the heights. There are faculties of the soul which one has only to rediscover in order to be connected in a waking dream (with the help of the frog who dives into the well) with these worlds far from earth. Here a sun-initiation is indicated, the way of a soul that seeks to make its way through to its eternal origin in the light. In fitting imaginations this fairy-tale reflects our descent to the earth. By night the frog clandestinely takes out both of the Sun-Daughter's eyes. Now she must follow him down to earth on the cobwebs, because only there can she get back her eyes from her bridegroom.

Here the mystery of man's becoming is indicated, for when the soul begins to live on earth she has to exchange her heavenly eyes for the bodily sense-organ. She has to go cosmically blind in order to awake to the earth.

Belief in the heavenly kernel of man's being — a belief which was common to all mankind and was radiated by the mysteries over all the continents of the earth — clearly ensouls the world of African fairy-tales. The Christ-light does not yet penetrate the African folk-mind, yet even there we find a very moving motif which is related to the Christian legend of the bishop who was fond of hunting that even on feast days he could not abandon his passion, until one day he encountered a stag with a golden cross between its antlers. The African story tells of a huntsman who follows a wounded animal up to a tree. Feeling tired, he lies down to rest and falls into a kind of waking dream. An old man takes him into the tree and leads him to a village filled with lamentation. In the chief's hut he sees the eldest son dying, shot through the breast. When he asks what has happened he is told that the villagers are all afraid of a huntsman who is killing their young men, although they have never harmed him. The huntsman realizes that he himself is meant. When he comes out of the tree he sees the animal lying before him, shot through the breast. From that day on he never touches a weapon. Going into the tree signifies that he is able to penetrate into the hidden regions of the realm of life. There he meets the group-soul of the animals he has been hunting.

Another well-known story is about the hare sent from the moon in earliest times to bring a comforting message to the people on earth: "Just as I am always renewed in death, so shall you also be renewed in death." But the hare does not believe it, so he tells the people: "The moon says that unlike himself, who in death is always renewed, you in death will not be renewed."

On hearing this the moon is very angry and hits the hare on the mouth so that his lip splits. When a Bushman looks at the hare's split lip, it should remind him that if anyone says death is the end of us, it is not true.

6. The Celtic heritage of wisdom

Celtic culture has had a pervasive influence on Western spiritual life. Though the national power of the Celts was broken by the Romans in the millennium before Christ, their influence worked on, fertilizing the Christian world of the Middle Ages with powerful spiritual and artistic impulses.

In Ireland, the Celtic heritage remained comparatively untouched until quite recent times. Belief and experience of elemental beings, "the good folk", still exists among the Irish people. They are conscious that these beings, though invisible to earthly eyes, are always present and participate in the life of man, helping and protecting, or playing tricks and taking revenge on anyone lacking respect for "the wee folk". They have a twilight character, sometimes inclined to good, sometimes activated by cunning and malice. We are told that they are angels who were cast out of heaven but have not sunk down to hell; they live now in the constant dread and uncertainty of whether or not they will receive grace at the last judgment.

From Ireland comes the elf-tale of "Little Foxglove". It is the story of a poor man from the Glen of Acherlow who, because of the big hump on his back, is avoided by people. He is mocked with the name "Little Foxglove" because he always wears a foxglove stalk in his little hat. The elves like to wear a red foxglove flower on their heads, and the Irish call them "Elfcaps".

One can imagine this poor man to be wise in the ways of nature; one who has great knowledge of healing herbs and magic and is at home with the elemental spirits. So in the moonlight, for that is the time when elves are most readily seen, he is permitted by them to enter an old dolmen, from which he hears coming the strange elfin music that so bewitches human beings. The elves take the hump off his back, for they come from the "Land of Youth" that knows no death.

The Grimms characterized the Irish fairy-tales in the following way: "Nothing could give a better picture of the Irishman's nature, always excitable, tinged with a certain wildness, and yet endowed with spiritual powers. Only such an agile imagination was capable of giving to the fundamental thought of the saga a narrative expression which constantly surprises us with new and unexpected turns. Nearly always the events become entangled or are unravelled by the intervention of one of the spirit beings who in count-less numbers inhabit water and land, wood and mountain, rock and wilderness, and who take on both the most charming and the ugliest forms. Heartless as they are, they seek to bind the human being to their circle, as if they harboured the desire to take into themselves his own warm life. People know their quirks and so keep out of their way, but try to stay on good terms with them."

One sees how light and darkness are mingled in these beings. In Nordic cosmology, which shares with the Celts a belief in elves, we find them divided into opposite kingdoms. The Edda distinguishes the light-elves who dwell in the world of the gods from the black-elves in the depths of the earth. By the latter are meant the dwarves.

The Celtic Renaissance brought about by the Irish poets and writers in the second half of the nineteenth century has helped resuscitate a long-buried spiritual heritage. This movement has been particularly effective in nurturing the seeds of a newly awakening spirituality, and ensuring man's survival in the midst of the flood of Western materialism. William Sharp, writing as Fiona Macleod at the turn of the century, expressed well the spirit of this renaissance.

The greatness of the Celtic race, that once extended from the British Isles across Gaul and Spanish Galicia through the whole of Central Europe and on down the Danube into the East, lay in the fact that it had known how to bring over a great spiritual heritage from sunken Atlantis. The Druids, that order of priestly wise men, controlled for a long period the spiritual education and guidance of the Celtic tribes. They were the faithful guardians of a service to the sun in which the wisdom of the Atlantean oracles worked on. This was an heirloom from ancient Hyperborea, preserved as a sacred heritage of the sun against the solidification of earth existence. It gave Celticism that special lustre which has flowed into many sagas and fairy-tales of the European peoples.

In this connection we may mention the Greeks. They spoke of a remarkable people, the Hyperboreans, in the land of the eternal sun that Apollo came from to journey to Hellas led by the swans. In Hellas he appeared at the Castalian Spring in Delphi. From Delphi, as the bestower of song and the teacher of the Muses, Apollo brought happiness to the nations.

This Greek myth refers to those mystery centres which guarded the secret of the unsullied origin of the human race, and guarded also the way to the source of eternal youth. It is told of Perseus, the Greek hero, that he first lived among the Hyperboreans and partook of their sacred repast before he was able to win his terrible battle with Medusa. Hercules had to reach the Hyperboreans when he wished to obtain the golden apples of the Hesperides. Many fairy-tales also reflect these impulses of the mysteries. They are to be found especially where a place is mentioned which is difficult to reach, and where abnormal trials have to be endured. The poets honoured in their songs the Hyperboreans to whom the way could not be found "neither by land nor by ship". This signifies that quite other ways are required in order to find entrance to their secrets: ways of spirit must be trod and ordeals of the soul passed through before the gates to that arcane revelation are opened. In the "Island of the Saints", where serpents cannot live — for such is said of Ireland — the holy places of Hibernia were the last guardians of the Hyperborean mysteries.

Against the background of the mystery-tradition of Hibernia we can now understand the Celtic mythology retold from the Gaelic by Ella Young. It tells of the descent of the high beings of the Sun, the De Danaans, to the green isle over which Brigit, the soul of the world, spreads her celestial mantle. In these mythical pictures we are shown a descent of the gods into Chaos as a sacrifice of the Sun-Powers to the world of darkness, for they come to bring order and beauty there. Here we can be reminded of the Manichaean outlook.

Ella Young came from Ireland, where she spent decades in villages and lonely settlements listening to these sagas. As an example we will quote only a few lines which tell of the founding of the exalted Sun-Oracle on the Hibernian Island: "Nuada, wielder of the White Light, set up the Spear of Victory in the centre of Ireland. It was like a great fiery fountain. It was like a singing flame. It burned continually, and from it every fire in Ireland was kindled."

This spear appears as the symbol of all the creative forces that are guarded by the sun-mystery and given to the surrounding world. In these places the secrets of white magic are administered. Then it is told how misshapen creatures, the Fomor, rise up out of the darkness and draw near to the circle of light that was formed over the island by the shining of the victorious spear. While they bask in this light they gradually absorb some of its power, and the desire grows in them to get the spear. In the end Balor, the one-eyed king of the Fomor, succeeds in doing this. The bearers of an ancient Atlantean element are always represented in sagas and fairy-tales as one-eyed. They are laggards in evolution; they still have the Cyclops' eye.

In the hands of these antagonists the spear of light is transformed into a fiery snake that fills the air around with demons. Thus the Fomor make themselves lords of the holy island and subjugate the people of light, the Dana. But the saga foretells the coming of an exalted sun-hero who will set up the holy spear again in the centre of Ireland before the end of the world comes. He is Lugh, who will break the power of darkness. This Perceval figure, as in the saga of the Grail, will bring back the holy spear to the sacred place.

In *Celtic Wonder Tales** in which Ella Young presents the heroic life of Fionn, we are told that when the world was young, before those radiant divine beings descended into the darkness of earth, they walked by the edge of the holy pool which is continually filled from the fountain of heaven. By its banks grow the holy hazel trees. Their topmost branches spread out into the invisible kingdoms. They bud and blossom and bear fruit all at the same time, and they let their glowing scarlet nuts fall one by one into the pool when they are ripe. Then the salmon, with scales that shine like sun-gold and moon-silver, rises up on mighty fins. He catches the nuts as they fall and swallows them. That is why he is so wise.

This "well of wisdom" never grows old; neither can the salmon tire, nor the holy hazels wither. Those who seek to reach the fountain of existence yearn to find this well and drink from it the wisdom that can make a man a seer. All true pictures reflected in the fairy-tales and myths come from this wisdom.

In the Grimms' tale of the "Hazel Branch" the Mother of God takes refuge from a viper that has sprung up out of the grass. It is said that hazel bushes offer the safest protection against vipers and snakes. It was therefore felt to be the opposite of this tree that is always represented with the serpent coiled round it — the tree from which Adam and Eve ate the fruit of knowledge which brought them death. The hazel appears as the picture of the Tree of Life on which grows the fruit of innocent wisdom. The hazelnut encloses its fruit in a hard shell — a picture of chastity. Now the apple, which in the fairy-tales stands for the fruit of the Tree of Knowledge, offers its flesh to view. When we behold the red-cheeked fruit we can feel how

---

* Reprinted Floris Books, Edinburgh 1985.

it tempts us to eat. Snow-White longs for the lovely apple but falls into a death-sleep when she eats the poisoned half. In the story of Cinderella, too, the hazel branch appears as a holy offshoot: the pious maiden plants it on her mother's grave and from it grows the tree on which the white dove settles, the dove that bestows heavenly clothing on the child.

The hazel-nuts that ripen on the Tree of Life do not offer a wisdom that can be lightly enjoyed. They are presented to the seeker after knowledge as riddles which cannot be solved without effort.

In her tales Ella Young brings saga-pictures from the most ancient Celtic store of wisdom. In them we can sense the sun-magic of a lost world which surges up again to the vision of the soul and which will be revealed in all its beauty in the future. As we read the message of these tales we can well understand what Padraic Colum meant when he said of the writer that she appeared to many of her acquaintances as a druidess, as one whom many a seeker in ancient Celtica would have found near the well into which the sacred hazelnuts fell, and from whom he would have learnt something of the mysteries.

Padraic Colum, who also belongs to the Celtic Renaissance, wrote *The King of Ireland's Son.** In this narrative a wealth of very ancient fairy-tale motifs and wonderful incidents are woven into a great saga of initiation undertaken by an Irish prince. One feels that this book is woven out of genuine imaginations, although as a whole it is the work of a modern writer.

The old "shanachies", the story-tellers and ballad singers of Ireland, were the guardians of such picture treasures, and thereby guardians of the folk-soul that thus remained conscious of a glorious past. Among

* Reprinted Floris Books, Edinburgh 1986.

such shanachies Colum grew up, often spending his
evenings sitting with them round peat-fires and listening to their tales. From this stream of folk-tradition he
drew the material for *The King of Ireland's Son* who
found the sword of light and passed through all the
trials which every true fairy-tale hero must undergo.

If we are to follow further the Celtic fairy-tale and saga
tradition, we must turn our attention to that tranquil
Breton world where so much that is significant in the
spiritual heritage of the Celts was able to take refuge.
In the fifth century large numbers of the original
Britons emigrated under pressure of the Anglo-Saxon
invasions. They settled in that north-western coastal
region of France which was formerly called Armorica
but which became known as Brittany. Here grew the
traditions which are linked with the legendary figure
of Arthur, last king of the Britons.

For these Britons Arthur was a symbol of all the
hopes of a glorious rebirth of the broken Celtic
heritage. In the twelfth century the figure of Arthur
became widely popular in Western Europe; the epic
poetry of the time did him honour, placing him in the
shining setting of the Round Table, with its famous
heroes. Now while the influence of the Druids
receded, or their best representatives were working
within Christianity, another order was called upon to
guard the national traditions and rekindle them as a
holy flame, an order which was able to preserve King
Arthur in his role of leader. This was the order of the
bards, who assembled in closed centres around their
bardic chairs. The ideals of chivalry in the Middle
Ages, as they lived and shone in the sagas that were
woven around the heroes of King Arthur's court, were
consciously elaborated and formed into verse by these
bards. This led to their taking on a supra-national

mission, while the national aspirations steadily declined. These ideals were incorporated in many of the figures of saga and fairy-tale which they had created with conscious intent and deeply implanted in the folk-mind.

But this Celtic spiritual heritage was fast dying away. Those with knowledge recognized that the times required quite new soul capabilities to maintain the connection with the spirit. In the fairy-tale figures of the simpleton these faculties emerged as saviours called upon by destiny.

The archetype of all those fortune-favoured fairy-tale heroes can be seen in the Breton fairy-tale of Peronnik.* He represents a precursor of Perceval, the hero of the Grail. "Per" indicates a disposition to penetrate or press on where others think they see impassable obstacles. Only souls that have not had their original powers stunted by intellectual upbringing and polite convention can get through the ordeals that the spirit-seeker is likely to encounter on his way.

As a wanderer who "had never learned any trade", and apparently quite unfit for any ordinary occupation, Peronnik wanders through Brittany. By chance he hears of the task which he feels he has strength to accomplish. After Peronnik has been well fed in the house of a peasant woman, a knight comes by and asks the way to the castle of Kerglas. He wants to win the golden bowl and the diamond lance which are hidden in a dark dungeon by the lord of the castle, the magician Rogéar. These two magical objects are worth more than all the crowns of the earth. The bowl brings unfailingly all the sustenance one could wish for. Whoever drinks from it will be healed of his pains and

* See *Breton Folk Tales*, G. Bell & Sons, London 1971.

the dead are brought to life if it touches their lips. But the diamond lance kills and destroys everything it strikes.

In the imaginations of the Grail these two objects play a decisive part. It is the holy vessel and the bleeding lance which appear to Perceval's soul-vision when he enters the castle in the evening. In the course of the story of the Grail the holy vessel and thebleeding lance are brought into a mystical connection with the sacrifice of Golgotha. In the fairy-tale of Peronnik this connection is still lacking; the confluence of the Grail stream, as cultivated among the Cathars, and the Arthur stream as the continuation of Celtic tradition, has not yet come about fully. Here we can see that twofold imagination without the mystical experiences of Christianity. Powers are indicated which work hidden in everyone although they escape the daytime consciousness completely. The two magical objects embrace a double mystery. One is hidden in that innocent life-process of our being which is regulated and maintained from the workings of the cosmos (in the imagination of the Grail, a maiden brings in the holy vessel). The other rises from the powerful urges which rage egotistically through the blood and are normally held in check by the waking consciousness (in the imagination of the Grail, the spear wounds the Fisher-King).

To gain possession of these valuable objects is to gain control over the hidden workings within our being. This appears to be impossible, for one would have to be able to penetrate the depths of sleep with a higher consciousness. The knight, however, has received instruction from a hermit. While Peronnik listens attentively, he describes the adventures that must be undertaken on the way to the magician's castle. There are seven ordeals, described pictorially. The knight can enumerate them, but only the "simpleton" succeeds in coming through them.

The fairy-tale says: "The strong try to meet danger with their strength and often perish in the attempt, but the weak try to get round things." The natural resourcefulness with which Peronnik prepares himself to attain his goal, and the presence of mind with which he manages to be master of every situation, are wonderfully described — as, for example, how he deals with the threatening lion from whom he must snatch the "laughing flower". Meeting the lion means perceiving our own heart-forces, with all their pride, irascibility and rebellion against the laws of destiny. Only when peace of heart has been established does the threatening lion become mild. This is not the place for violence. Peronnik does not fight with the lion lest he goad him to extremes. He knows how to engage the lion with his foolery. Humour is a sign of the freedom that one can win over oneself. To attain it is to be able to pluck the laughing flower. Only with this flower can the simpleton, after defeating the magician, open the passage to the inner vault of the castle in which the golden bowl and the diamond lance are hidden. If the depths are to be opened in which the mysteries of life are protected against any impure seizure, a soul-power of plantlike purity must blossom.

Equipped with the two magical objects, the victor goes to the court of the King of Brittany at Nantes. When Peronnik arrives he finds the town under siege and everybody starving. In this predicament the king proclaims that the city's deliverer shall be his heir. With the diamond lance Peronnik strikes down his enemies, and with the life-giving bowl he restores the fallen to life. He goes through the world as a liberator and bestower of blessings. In the end the fairy-tale sends him off on a crusade to free the Holy Land from the Saracens. In this way a twist is given to the story: in Peronnik arises a hero of Christendom who is able to lead it to victory and even bring reconciliation with the infidels. The cosmopolitan spirit of the saga of the Grail is already being breathed into the fairy-tale.

This attitude of world-citizenship comes to meet us also in the Breton fairy-tale of the "Crystal Palace". It tells of a journey to the mysteries in which the simpleton — here called Yvon, who is seeking his beautiful sister, Yvonne — braves every danger as he goes east to a crystal palace on the far shore of the Black Sea. This is a journey into the kingdom beyond the threshold of death. All the trials indicate this, especially the silence that is practised in that crystal realm. For this is the behaviour the soul must perfect in its communion with the dead. The fairy-tale embraces also a knowledge of that mystery centre "on the far shore of the Black Sea" which spirit-seekers have known from olden times. It is the same one to which the Argonauts undertook their voyage and whose fame had reached the West.

On a final note we would mention a Gaelic fairy-tale which bears the stamp of that comprehensive cosmopolitan orientation which has always marked the Celtic tradition. This is the "Celtic Dragon Myth", a fairy-tale told among the Gaels in many variations. For the comprehensive nature of this fairy-tale the name is too onesided, for it can be considered as a whole compendium of fairy-tale motifs, embracing in harmony the various ways that lead to the spirit.

It is similar to the great fairy-tale of the "Two Brothers" in Grimms' collection, which tells of two brothers whose ways part, but who find each other again in the end when one goes to aid the other. The

Gaelic fairy-tale tells of three brothers who go forth into the world: the first east, the second takes the middle way, and the third goes west. They are the sons of an old smith who becomes a fisherman. At first he is a poor fisherman living by the sea-shore and catching nothing. But he becomes rich through the intervention of a mermaid. He promises his eldest son to her in return for good fishing. The fisherman appears in many fairy-tales, and the saga of the Grail also tells of the rich fisherman. He lives on the borders of the two realms and will one day be able to carry over revelations of the spirit from the night into earth-consciousness.

What is now told is related in its ground-motifs to the fairy-tale of the "Golden Children". The fisherman catches a talking fish. This happens three times. Then the fish tells him to cut him up in a particular way and give his wife a piece of the heart and liver to eat; then she will bear him three boys.

When the three sons turn fourteen, they want to journey into the world. The father forges an iron rod for the eldest to give him mighty strength for his journey. These are thought-forces that are beginning to awaken in the youth: with them he will overcome giants and will finally win the fight with the dragon that will free the king's daughter. When he wins her hand, he inherits a kingdom. The fairy-tale calls it Greece, for his way leads him to the East. Because his father is trying to keep him away from the mermaid to whom he was pledged from his birth, he has to avoid going anywhere near salt water.

This spirit-seeker goes the way travelled by the peoples who wandered from Atlantis to the East. They sought the mainland. All dreamlike clairvoyance that drew men into dialogue with the elemental powers had to die away in them. They had to master the realm of the giants: in clear thought-power the soul was to find the spirit. At one time Perseus had to win the fight with the dragon in order to free the maiden. By the legendary figure of Perseus the Greeks signified the great king who built Mycenae: he ranks as the founder of that Greek culture which was the first to take on the mission of clear thinking and so was able to fight for the freedom of the personality.

The second son, who chose the middle way, comes to the court of a king where there are no women except for the king's daughter who is kept hidden in a tower. He reaches her in the form of a dove and wins her after accomplishing the tasks set before him. Here is out-lined the way of a mystic, indeed of a Christian mystic, as a closer examination of the motifs shows. When the story says that he wins the daughter of the King of France, it acknowledges that in the early Middle Ages France had become the centre from which radiated esoteric Christianity.

The third brother rides westward, where all ways lead to the sea. His ordeals are of a quite different character. At night he enters a deserted castle. A lantern with a candle in it comes to meet him and leads him on through the dark rooms. The king's daughter in this enchanted castle remains invisible to him at first. He can free her only if he passes the test of being near her without touching her. Only when the senses are silent can the spirit gradually begin to communi-cate itself in its true form. Thus after manifold trials he wins the daughter of the king of the golden kingdom of which he shall sometime be king.

On this way one has to do with an awakening in the realm of night. A light that begins to shine in the darkness becomes the guide in those hidden regions where the Hyperborean mysteries are kept locked away from a mankind caught in the consciousness of the senses. The Celtic tradition knows that this sun-bright realm of the spirit must be found again if man is not to lose his connection with the powers of his origin. The other brothers are finally turned to stone by wicked magic and only the third brother, who has won the king's daughter of the golden castle (she is the same as the princess whom the king's son in "Faithful Johannes" sets out to win), is able to come to their aid. He will be their awakener, although at first they do not understand his deed and resent it. But few narrators know how to tell in what way the great reconciliation between the brothers will come about. The final harmonization of the three streams seems not yet willing to reveal itself completely. The question remains, when and how it will come to pass. It is a question for mankind whether the world wanderers who have spread out to the East, the Middle and the West will come to know each other as brothers again.

It also concerns the awakening of the peoples of the earth to the spirit. The Celtic soul is full of prophecy. It believes that the great figures of ancient times will arise again among men when the hour strikes and the world in its need begins to search for the lost original wisdom. Thus the bards foretold that Arthur shall come again and gather his knights around him to set up the kingdom of the spirit. The Irish story-tellers point to the figure of Fionn, whom they see as the last of the heroes who attained to the mysteries. They wait upon his return. Our examination of the fairy-tales would end upon a final note of such expectation:

> Fionn, the light one, from the well
> Where'er with sacred branches decked
> The hazel-nut trees downward bend
> Hath all world-wisdom won.

Now hidden "neath green grassy knoll,
On royal throne in hall of rock,
His spirit waits horn's thunder blast
That calls him forth to save.

An ancient yet eternal child
Resplendent in his virtue's gleam
He breaks the darkness of the times
And summons youth to wake.

Index

Names of stories are in *italics*

The Young Child

*Creative Living with
two to four-year-olds*

Daniel Udo de Haes

Behind the dreamy, astonished or delighted eyes of the little child are hidden depths of experience which we adults can barely grasp. The author accepts the pre-earthly origin of the child in its full reality. He shows how the little child, still close to the sphere of his origin, perceives something of the cosmic in his environment: a ball awakens a slumbering memory of the spheres of the cosmos. And why should a toddler wish to build a "house"? Sounds and gestures remind the child of a language greater than his own.

It is of the greatest importance that we do not try to awaken the child too early from his dreams of pre-earthly life. Out of his wealth of experience as a father, grandfather, and teacher, the author traces the stages of development and suggest suitable activities which will strengthen the child for the world in which he is to live.

Floris Books
Anthroposophic Press